# THE
# Arthritis Foundation's
## *guide to*
# PAIN
# Management

## SUSAN BERNSTEIN

Chief Medical Editor
John H. Klippel, MD

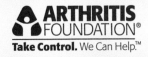

AN OFFICIAL PUBLICATION
OF THE ARTHRITIS FOUNDATION

Published by
Arthritis Foundation
1330 West Peachtree Street
Atlanta, GA 30309

Printed in the United States

———————————

1st Printing 2003

Library of Congress Card Catalog Number:
2003100376

ISBN: 0-912423-39-0

Editorial Director: SUSAN BERNSTEIN

Creative Director: AUDREY GRAHAM

Art Director: TRACIE BULLIS

Production Artist: JILL DIBLE

## ACKNOWLEDGEMENTS

*The Arthritis Foundation's Guide to Pain Management* is written for people in chronic pain. Among this population are many of the 70 million Americans who have arthritis or other related diseases. The causes of chronic pain are numerous and varied. This book was created to help people in pain understand the nature of their pain, and to make sense of the many medical and alternative treatments available.

Bringing *The Guide to Pain Management* to completion was a team effort, including the significant contributions of dedicated physicians, health-care professionals, Arthritis Foundation volunteers, writers, editors, designers and Arthritis Foundation staff.

The author of the book is Susan Bernstein, Director of Book Development and Acquisition at the Arthritis Foundation. She is also the author of the Arthritis Foundation's books *Tips for Good Living With Arthritis* and *Change Your Life: Simple Strategies to Lose Weight, Get Fit and Improve Your Outlook*. The art director of the book is Audrey Graham, Arthritis Foundation Creative Director. The book's production design and cover design was done by Jill Dible.

The medical editor of the book was John H. Klippel, MD, Medical Director of the Arthritis Foundation and former clinical director of the National Institute of Arthritis and Musculoskeletal and Skin Diseases (NIAMS), a component of the National Institutes of Health. Dr. Klippel currently serves on the editorial boards of several medical journals, and is a Visiting Professor of Internal Medicine at the Johns Hopkins University. He is a diplomat of the American Board of Internal Medicine, board-certified in rheumatology, and a fellow of the American College of Physicians and the American College of Rheumatology.

The Arthritis Foundation would like to acknowledge the contributions of the following people who served as reviewers of the book prior to publication, and thank them for their efforts on behalf of the Arthritis Foundation:

Daniel J. Clauw, MD, Professor of Medicine, Division of Rheumatology, and Director, Chronic Pain and Fatigue Research Center; Interim Director, Center for the Advancement of Clinical Research; University of Michigan, Ann Arbor, Mich., and a member of the American College of Rheumatology

Doris K. Cope, MD, Staff Member of the University of Pittsburgh Medical Center and the St. Margaret Pain Medicine Center, University of Pittsburgh Physicians, Department of Anesthesiology, in Pittsburgh, Penn., and a member of the American Society of Anesthesiologists' committee on pain medicine

John E. Tetzlaff, MD, Head of the Section of Acute Perioperative Care and Director of the Center for Anesthesiology Education of the Division of Anesthesiology and Critical Care Medicine at The Cleveland Clinic Foundation in Cleveland, Ohio, and a member of the American Society of Anesthesiologists' committee on pain medicine

Carolyn Amisano of Suwanee, Ga., a volunteer who has had rheumatoid arthritis for 28 years, who reviewed the book from the perspective of the person living with chronic pain

**The mission of the Arthritis Foundation is to improve lives through leadership in the prevention, control and cure of arthritis and related diseases.**

# Contents

# Contents *continued*

# FOREWORD

Chronic pain is an enormous problem that affects millions of people each day. Pain affects their ability to do their jobs, puts a strain on their personal relationships, keeps them from getting a good night's sleep, and, in some cases, causes disability. While acute pain can put you out of commission for a few days or weeks, chronic pain lingers for months, years, or sadly for many people, a lifetime. For many people, pain simply takes over their lives, and interferes with almost every daily activity.

There are many causes of chronic pain: Arthritis, back pain, fibromyalgia, injuries and many more. Currently, more than 70 million Americans – that is almost one in four – lives with arthritis or a related disease. Arthritis is a major cause of chronic pain and the nation's number one cause of disability. Yet, there is great hope for people who suffer from pain, whether it is caused by arthritis or another condition. There is hope because virtually all forms of pain can be better managed by a decision to take control of your pain.

The road to managing pain begins with figuring out what's causing the problem and understanding what you can do about it. Diagnosis can be quick or can take weeks or months, requiring patience and commitment from you and your doctor. Once a diagnosis is made, you must work with your doctor to find effective treatments for your pain. With new advances in pain medicine, there is much that can be done in the way of medications, exercises, preventive behavior and surgery that can be used to treat pain so that you to get on with your life. Medical research has produced new, technologically advanced methods for treating chronic pain, many of which are described in this book. In addition, many people with chronic pain can turn to *complementary therapies* – treatments for pain that exist in conjunction with their medical therapies – to ease pain or the stress that often accompanies it.

It is important that you learn from your episodes of pain. In many cases, you can prevent or at least mitigate pain through simple lifestyle changes. This book, *The Arthritis Foundation's Guide to Pain Management,* gives you the tools you need to understand your pain and develop a plan for managing its effects on a daily basis. In these pages, you will learn about the most common causes of chronic pain, their many symptoms, how your doctor will make a diagnosis and how you will work with your health-care professional to begin a course of treatment.

Most importantly, you will learn how your actions will impact your health – from exercise to diet to stress and pain management. This book will help you take control of chronic pain – instead of allowing the pain to take control of your life.

The Arthritis Foundation believes that the actions you take to control your chronic pain play a large and important role in determining your outcome. Education about your condition, self-management, and taking personal responsibility are tools of empowerment and keys to achieving control of chronic pain. This book, *The Arthritis Foundation's Guide to Pain Management,* is a practical and clear guide that will hopefully help you achieve a healthier, more fulfilling life.

John H. Klippel, MD
Medical Director
Arthritis Foundation

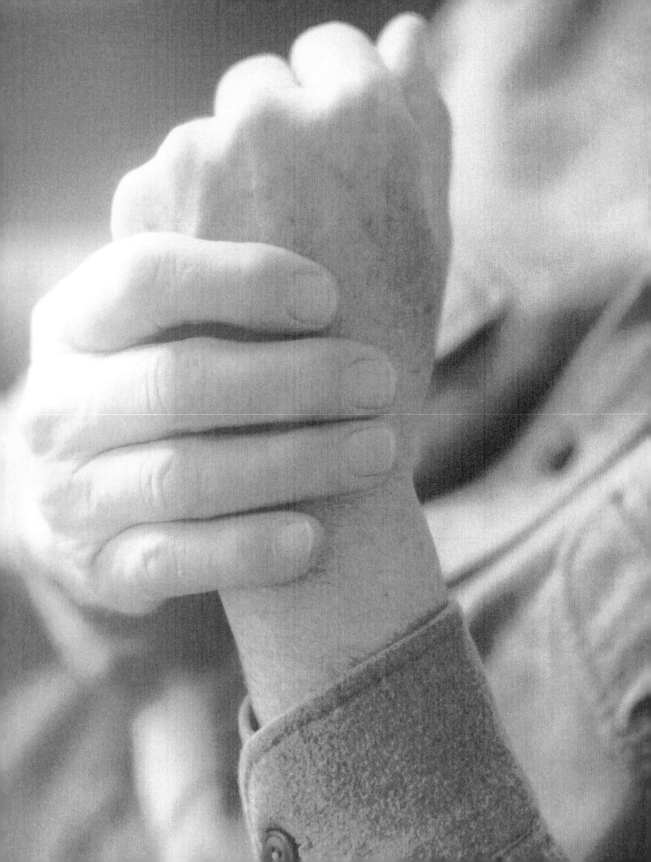

# Introduction

**Pain,** (pān) *n.*, A sensation of hurting, or strong discomfort, in some part of the body, caused by an injury, disease, or functional disorder, and transmitted through the nervous system.

*Webster's New World Dictionary, Third College Edition*

Pain, as the dictionary defines it, seems like a simple matter. You feel hurt or uncomfortable when you have had an injury or illness. When you are experiencing pain, however, trying to describe how it feels, pinpoint its cause or find a helpful treatment are anything but easy.

Pain is one of the most common health complaints among people today. There are many different types of pain: A dull ache, a sharp stab, a recurring throb, a sudden sting, a constant burning, and many more. Pain may be caused by any number of ailments, including disease, injuries, stress and others. But a few facts are common when discussing any type of pain or any of pain's causes. Here are the important points to remember as you begin reading this book:

- Pain is real.
- Pain has a cause.
- Pain can impair your ability to perform your everyday activities.
- Pain is treatable.
- Pain can, in most cases, be managed.

There are many different ways to treat your pain, including new methods developed by recent medical research. However, treating pain can be a complicated process for doctors and patients. Some people may struggle to find the most effective treatment for their type of pain, particularly if they have *chronic* or long-lasting pain. Others may find relief from their pain, but suffer from unpleasant or life-disrupting side effects from pain-fighting or *analgesic* medications. In addition to drugs and other medical devices to treat pain, there are many lifestyle changes – a practice known as *self-management* – people may make to help relieve and prevent pain. These changes may include exercise, getting proper rest, controlling stress or curbing drinking alcohol or smoking.

Because there are so many different causes and types of pain, and so many methods to alleviate pain, some physicians actually specialize in treating pain itself. These professionals practice in a field known as *pain medicine.* Yet you are most likely to receive attention and treatment for your pain from your primary-care doctor, such as an internist or family physician. Or, if you have a serious chronic illness, such as arthritis or fibromyalgia, you might receive pain treatment from the specialist (like a *rheumatologist*, a doctor with specialized training in treating arthritis-related diseases) who treats you for this illness.

As we noted earlier, there are many health problems that can cause intense pain. This pain may be *acute* (serious, but lasting for a short time) or chronic. But this book will mainly focus on causes of chronic pain and treatments for that pain, including drugs, surgery, alternative therapies, supplements and things you can do on your own, like exercise or stress-relief techniques.

Why is chronic pain uniquely challenging? Acute pain, such as that caused by a broken bone, an ear infection or a kidney stone, can be excruciating. Yet acute pain can often be easily managed with medications, ice application, elevation and rest. Once the injury or health problem that caused the acute pain has healed, the pain usually is gone. But chronic pain, such as that caused by arthritis, is a daily occurrence. The pain may subside at times, and get suddenly worse at other times (an experience known as a *flare*), but it is always present in the person's life.

The most important first step in treating your pain is making an appointment with your doctor. Remember: Pain is not something you "just have to live with." Your pain has a cause – something that may be a serious health problem that needs to be addressed and treated with medications and, possibly, surgery – and should be diagnosed by a doctor. Don't try to treat serious pain on your own.

In some cases, *over-the-counter* medicines can be used to treat your mild pain. But for most people with chronic pain, or even a severe flare of pain that is usually manageable, the best option is to see a doctor. You and your doctor will create a *pain-management plan*. With this plan, you and your doctor can start treating your pain now and keep it from getting worse.

What happens if you just "live with the pain"? Pain that continues without proper treatment affects your whole body. Your muscles might weaken, you can have stomach problems, your immune system (your body's way of healing itself) can suffer, or you can become depressed. It's important that you treat your pain, and your doctor can help you.

Your doctor may not just prescribe medicine, but also suggest treatments like heat or cold therapy, exercises, a brace or splint, and others. We will discuss all of these treatments and many more in this book. You should use this information to add to the discussions you have with your doctor – but never as a replacement for a doctor's advice and treatment.

Whether you have arthritis, fibromyalgia, bursitis or another form of recurring or chronic pain, your doctor can prescribe treatments for your pain. He may also prescribe treatments for the disease that is causing your pain. In other words, some powerful drugs modify the processes in the body that cause the inflammation that may be causing your pain. By treating the disease, your symptoms, including pain, can be alleviated.

Your doctor can provide powerful tools to fight your pain and the problems that cause it. Yet there is much that you can do on your own to control and, in some cases, prevent your pain. The person with a chronic illness must learn ways to self-manage their ongoing pain through a combination of medications and lifestyle changes. While it is not necessary for you to just live with the pain or "grin and bear it," it is necessary for you to live your life and avoid the negative consequences of chronic pain. It's that mental challenge – keeping your spirits up, avoiding negativity and focusing on something other than your pain – that can be the most difficult to achieve.

This book will outline a number of strategies to relieve pain. Some strategies are medical and others involve alternative approaches to drugs and other medical methods. Some-thing as simple as a daily stretching routine or applying a bag of ice cubes or frozen peas can help alleviate some pain. This book also contains a chapter on strategies to reduce stress (which can worsen pain) and use your mind's power to help fight pain.

*The Arthritis Foundation's Guide to Pain Management* will offer you a great deal of information about pain and the latest ways to keep pain in control. By working with your doctor and exploring some of the strategies in this book, you hopefully will find the methods that help you. The Arthritis Foundation's intention in creating this book is to help guide you to effective methods of beating your pain, so you can live the full, active life you deserve.

Don't let pain win this battle! We can help you take control of your pain and start living well once more.

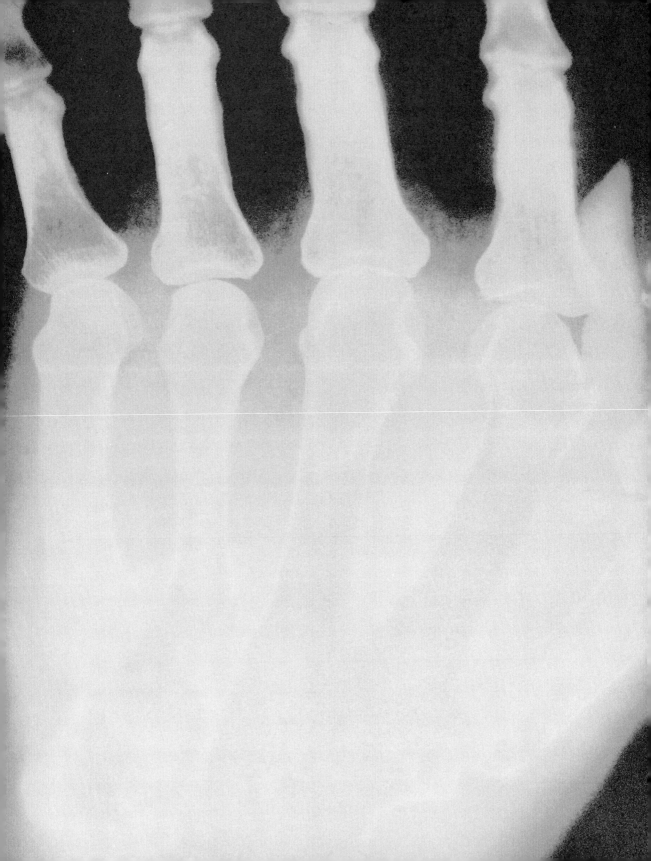

# What Is Pain?

---

1

# CHAPTER 1: WHAT IS PAIN?

Pain is not just a problem in and of itself. Pain is a *symptom*. Pain is the body's warning system. It's a signal from your body that something is wrong – just like a security alarm that buzzes when something goes awry. For example, if you step on a thumbtack, it is important to stop walking and remove the tack from your foot. Pain is the body's signal that you need to take action. You can treat the pain itself, but it's also important to know what may be causing the pain.

While pain that only lasts a short time may be treated and then mostly forgotten, chronic or long-lasting pain – like the pain associated with arthritis, fibromyalgia, chronic back problems and similar diseases – is an alarm that keeps ringing and ringing. You feel that the pain is always there, subsiding at times and suddenly worsening at others. Pain is not only a nuisance; it also may be a clear message from your body that something is wrong. The problem causing your pain should be addressed or the pain may worsen. If you ignore the pain, the cause of the pain may progress.

If you are in pain, you are not alone. Millions of Americans experience some kind of pain on a regular basis, and many of these people experience chronic or long-lasting pain. This category of pain, which includes the pain of arthritis, has a tremendous impact on the lives of those who have it. According to the American Pain Foundation, the cost of treating chronic pain, including medical expenses, lost income from days out of work, and lost productivity on the job due to workers' sick leave, is at billions of dollars per year.

What's more, chronic pain can be very difficult to control or treat. According to the Arthritis Foundation's publication *Speaking of Pain,* only 43 of 100 people surveyed who report having moderate to severe pain said they had a "great deal of control" over that pain. The same report stated that only 42 percent of those surveyed say their doctor completely understood their pain. So communicating your pain to your doctor, understanding it yourself and finding the right treatments to control the pain are key.

Each person experiences pain differently. For one person, a headache might be an annoying interruption to the workday, while another person might spend hours in bed with a cold washcloth on her forehead. Why? The intensity and nature of the first person's headache might be quite different from the headache experienced by the second person.

In addition, each person's unique psychological and physical composition – as well as gender, age and even cultural background, according to some researchers – may have an effect on how he or she perceives pain. This variance makes it even more difficult for health-care professionals to assess your pain and pinpoint the correct treatments.

There are many reasons for pain, and different categories and types of pain. In this chapter, we'll learn more about how pain happens, why it occurs and what physical problems may lead to serious pain.

To begin to understand why you feel pain, you must first understand an elaborate network in your body: the *nervous system*. The nervous system, masterminded by its boss, the brain, runs every process in your body, from feeling to breathing to digesting food. Without it, you would be just a lump of flesh. The nervous system brings you to life and action. It governs every movement in your body, including those you are aware of (picking up a leaf and feeling its surface) and those you rarely notice (your heartbeat or your breathing).

The nervous system is made up of two subsystems: the *central nervous system,* which includes your brain and spinal cord, and the *peripheral nervous system,* which includes all the little nerves stretching throughout the rest of your body. Nerves are fibrous tissues that sense all kinds of stimuli. As noted above, they regulate and run different processes in your body. There are three main kinds of nerves:

- **Autonomic nerves** regulate normal body functions such as heart rate, breathing, sweating, blood pressure and digestion of food.
- **Motor nerves** regulate the motion of your muscles, allowing you to move your hands and feet, walk, sit, stand and perform other functions.
- **Sensory nerves** are the nerves that feel, allowing you to sense texture, temperature and pressure, as well as sensations such as pleasure or pain.

Some nerve fibers have highly sensitive *nerve endings,* also known as *nociceptors,* which are specialized in feeling various types of stimuli. Some of these nerve endings perceive pain. On the following pages, we'll learn more about this system and how you feel pain.

## HOW PAIN HAPPENS

Pain, as we said earlier, is almost like a fire alarm ringing in your body. As in a fire, a smoke detector may sense a fire in your house. It begins buzzing, and sends a distress signal to the 911 center, where an emergency operator takes the call. The operator then sends a quick message to the nearest fire station, which dispatches a ready crew to splash water on the fire, bring the situation under control if possible, and assess the damage done.

When you feel pain, what you are really experiencing is an elaborate communication and response effort that's similar to a monitored fire alarm system. Only in place of smoke detectors, alarms and 911 operators are the important players within your body: the nerves, the spinal cord and the brain.

In your body, the smoke detector is an elaborate network of millions of strands of nerves around your body. Nerves are located all over your skin, in your bones, joints and muscles, and even around internal organs like your stomach or liver. The miniscule fibers wind together into cords, and these cords wind all over the body to allow you to feel various sensations. The specialized endings of the fibers are called *receptors,* and they change physical and chemical signals into messages in the nervous system.

Different nerves have different functions – some sense pain, others pleasure, others cold, pressure, heat and more. Some nerve endings sense the presence of *inflammation*, or swelling, that is often a symptom of arthritis. These nerves coursing throughout your body are known as the peripheral nerves. Receptors that sense the harmful events that cause pain are called nociceptors. Sensitive nerve endings, the nociceptors are part of this peripheral nervous system.

Nociceptors are tiny: it takes more than 1,000 nociceptors to cover an area of your skin the size of a postage stamp. There are more nociceptors in some parts of your body than others, which is why some areas of your body are more sensitive than others. Your skin and exposed membranes like your eyes have far more concentrated amounts of nerve endings. Body parts like muscles and bones, protected beneath your skin, have a fewer nociceptors, and the coverings of your internal organs have even fewer. Chronic pain felt in your bones, joints and muscles can be strong even though there are fewer nerve endings there than in highly sensitive areas like the tips of your fingers.

## How Nerves Call 911

Your nerve endings transmit feelings by sending electrical impulses through the body and up the *spinal cord*, the network of nerves running up and down the spine in your back to your brain. The spinal cord acts almost like the telephone system in your town. The nerves in the spinal cord are involved in a process like your body's version of a 911 emergency telephone call. The brain is the command center of the body. It receives the electrical messages, process the information sent by the nerves, and delivers orders to other body parts to react accordingly.

In other words, if you touch a hot stove accidentally, the nerves in your fingers may sense a sharp burning. But you feel the burning only after your nerves send a signal to the brain that this is occurring and your brain sends a message back to your fingers that the stove is hot and your skin hurts from the burn. (Don't worry. The process moves very quickly!) Your brain tells you that you feel pain and to react by pulling your finger away. Like that 911 operator, your brain takes in the distress signal and dispatches the appropriate responses to the problem. The first response it sends back to the fingers is the feeling of pain – if you didn't feel the pain, you wouldn't pull your hand away and it would burn. While the pain messages for acute and chronic pain are sent at the same rate, you might become aware of acute pain in an instant – it's like a sudden shock. Chronic pain, which you feel over and over again, day in and day out, may be something you try to become accustomed to.

Does every message sent by the nerve endings get to the brain? Not necessarily. Sometimes, damage to the nerve endings from certain diseases or injuries can keep you from feeling pain. That's a dangerous situation, because the pain messages your brain receives allow it to make adjustments to preserve your health. However, there are some ways that your body can filter pain messages to the brain to help control your pain without putting your health and life in danger.

## The Gate Theory of Pain

So when nociceptors sense something harmful is happening to their part of the body, they send electrical messages up the spinal cord to the brain. But before those messages can reach the brain, they have to go through special nerves in the spinal cord that control which pain messages move to the brain and which ones will not. This concept is what is known as the "gate control" theory of pain, and these nerve cells act as one set of tiny but powerful "gatekeepers" of the pain process.

If you touch a red-hot log in the fireplace and burn your hand, causing severe, acute pain that signals a possible danger to your body, the theory holds that your gatekeeper nerve cells will open the "pain gate" wide to let the signals pass through quickly. Your brain receives the impulses and sends a quick message back to the various nerves in the hand to feel the pain and pull away.

In contrast, some pain messages that are weaker and do not indicate danger to the body, such as a little flea bite or a minor scratch, may not get through the pain gate or may pass slowly to the brain. You might not be aware of them at first, and your awareness of the discomfort might grow gradually rather than be felt immediately.

The gate theory is one hypothesis about how you feel pain. Some experts now consider pain a more complex, ongoing process, particularly where chronic pain is concerned.

Pain signals must cross a gap, called a *synapse*, between each nerve on their way to the brain. How do these signals cross the gap? The first nerve cell secretes a special chemical called a *neurotransmitter*, which spreads across the gap and contacts receptor sites on the second nerve. The neurotransmitter causes a change to happen to the surface of the second cell and creates an electrical signal.

After this journey, the neurotransmitter either breaks down or returns to the first nerve. There are many different types of neurotransmitters, including *serotonin*. Scientists believe that serotonin plays a role in the release of chemicals like endorphins, which can block the transmission of pain signals across synapses and temporarily relieve pain. Opiate drugs mimic the body's natural chemicals for a similar result.

Is the pain process different in people with chronic pain? Scientists now believe it is, a theory called *neuroplasticity*. According to this theory, continuous pain stimuli may cause nerve cells to change their structure and behavior. More neurotransmitters may be released and the process of pain signal transmission may alter. Nerve cells may develop a "memory of pain," leading to heightened sensitivity to even small sensations. Analgesic or pain-killing drugs like acetaminophen (*Tylenol*) or *opiates* (such as codeine) can alter the pain-perception processes in the spinal cord and the brain so you feel less pain.

Endorphins and similar body chemicals called *enkephalins*, both produced in the brain and spinal cord, have the ability to attach to the gatekeepers and block pain transmission.

While the body can produce its own painkilling substances, it can also produce too much of other substances that can cause pain. Some people may produce abnormally high levels of a chemical called *substance P*. At unusually high levels, substance P can intensify the pain messages sent to the brain, widening the pain gate. Researchers believe that people with fibromyalgia, a disease marked by chronic muscle pain and heightened pain sensitivity, may produce too much substance P.

What else can a person do to fight the pain response? What if the brain receives other sensations in addition to the pain messages? If you were to walk by a doorway and accidentally bump your elbow against the frame, it would hurt. The nerve endings in your elbow would sense the bump, send pain messages to the brain, and your brain would send back the impulse to feel the pain. If you rubbed or massaged the elbow, your brain would then receive messages from nerve endings of a soothing pressure. These new sensation messages would, in effect, speak over the pain messages, blocking their transmission and lessening their impact in the brain.

## The Command Center

How do pain messages actually turn into the pain you feel? When cells experience some type of damage – either due to injury or disease – the cells release chemicals into the bloodstream, such as cytokines, prostaglandins, serotonin, histamines and more. When the system works properly, the chemicals released send messages to the brain. All of these chemicals play roles in how the body reacts to danger, triggering pain, inflammation, raised body temperature or

other responses once they reach the brain. In some cases, the chemicals don't act as they should, and pain, inflammation or other responses are out of control. In these cases, some drugs or other therapies may help suppress certain out-of-control body chemicals.

When pain messages pass through the pain gate to your brain, they first come to the brain's processing facility, the *thalamus*. The thalamus sorts and prioritizes pain messages and then sends them on to two other parts of the brain for processing: the *cerebral cortex* and the *limbic center*. It is only when the messages reach these parts of the brain that you actually *feel* pain. As we said earlier, the entire process usually happens in an instant, so you are unaware of the complicated journey of the sensation.

Your cerebral cortex is the part of your brain that creates thoughts. The cerebral cortex receives messages and decides how to react to pain. In other words, it may tell you to pull your hand away from a red-hot stove burner. But the cerebral cortex also governs those autonomic nerves we learned about earlier. These nerves regulate many involuntary body functions, such as temperature, blood pressure and others. So if you stepped on a nail, your cerebral cortex would send messages to your foot to feel the pain and prompt you to pull your foot off the nail, but it also would send messages to the autonomic nerves to send necessary blood and nutrients to the site of the wound. In cases of sustained pain, the cerebral cortex might order the release of endorphins from other parts of the brain to help suppress the pain.

Pain messages also go to the limbic center of the brain, where emotional responses are created. Pain messages may elicit a response of fear or worry from the limbic center. The limbic center of the brain can have an effect on how you perceive the pain, making it seem more intense or less so.

## DIFFERENT TYPES OF PAIN

As we learned earlier, there are two types of pain: acute and chronic. Your doctor may use these terms when you see him or her for treatment. Acute pain lasts for only a short time, but it can be sharply painful. Chronic means that the pain may go on and on. Your doctor may use other terms to describe your pain that could be confusing, so we'll try to explain them.

### Nociceptive Pain

Nociceptive pain is pain sensed by those tiny nerves that run throughout the body and the surfaces of muscles, organs and joints. Often, nociceptive pain is caused by injuries to tissues in the body like muscles, ligaments, tendons, bones, joints, skin or other organs. Arthritis and even an injury from a car accident are examples. Nociceptive pain often feels like aching, throbbing or a long-lasting soreness. Some doctors think that nociceptive pain, if it persists, also can cause problems in your nerves and spinal cord, altering how they function in the pain process. If your nociceptors keep sending pain message after pain message through the "alarm system," you might feel pain all the time, even when there is nothing really wrong.

### Neuropathic Pain

Pain that comes when nerves are injured or inflamed is *neuropathic pain*. This kind of pain can happen anywhere in your body, because nerves run throughout your body. Some causes of neuropathic pain are accidents or injuries, back problems that involve damaged or compressed nerves, or even nerve-damaging drugs for treating major illnesses like cancer. Often, neuropathic pain feels like a burning sensation or a shooting pain.

### Idiopathic Pain

Also called chronic pain of complex etiology, *idiopathic pain* is a term for painful conditions that don't fall into one of the two previous categories. Sometimes, doctors don't know (or don't yet know) the internal mechanisms that cause these painful problems, but the pain is very real for those who have them. Doctors use terms such as chronic pain of complex etiology or non-nociceptive pain to describe the pain of fibromyalgia, migraine headaches, temporomandibular joint disorder (TMD or sometimes called TMJ), irritable bowel syndrome, myofascial pain, chronic low-back pain or atypical chest pain. (We'll learn more about some of these conditions later in the book.) Because their doctors cannot readily identify a clear physical cause of the pain, people with these disorders often cannot find proper treatment or relief. People with this type of pain may find it difficult to communicate the nature of their pain to their doctors also, creating more obstacles to pain relief. Chronic emotional stress may trigger these painful conditions in part, or it may make it worse.

Pain can have a major impact on your ability to have a normal, fulfilling life. We're not talking about short-lived pain from a broken ankle or an ear infection. While such acute pain can be severe, it lasts for a few days and can be treated effectively.

In contrast, chronic pain, like that caused by arthritis, fibromyalgia, gout, lupus, back pain, tendinitis or similar diseases can prevent you from doing or enjoying basic activities. It can keep you from working, taking care of your home and your family, doing your daily chores or participating in leisure activities.

Pain can be a major cause of *disability* for some people with chronic diseases like arthritis. Disability is a term that means the lack of ability to work or take care of yourself without help. People whose pain worsens to the point where they experience disability may have to apply for government assistance or depend heavily on family or loved ones for help. Your doctor will work with you to determine the impact pain is having on your ability to function by measuring your pain on various charts and talking to you about what activities you can no longer do. We'll talk more about these methods in Chapter Two.

## ARTHRITIS: A MAJOR CAUSE OF CHRONIC PAIN

Arthritis is a major cause of chronic pain, affecting as many as 70 million, or one in three, American adults. It is the leading cause of disability in the United States. Arthritis symptoms include pain that can range from mild and occasional to terrible and persistent, as well as swelling, fatigue and impaired movement.

Why does arthritis cause so much pain and so many problems for so many people? One reason is that arthritis pain is long-lasting and often degenerative – it can worsen as the person's disease progresses. Arthritis can often be systemic, affecting other parts of the body besides joints. Because of their arthritis pain, many people stop exercising or doing much movement at all, causing their muscles to shrink and *atrophy*, becoming weaker. Lack of exercise can contribute to other health problems, such as obesity and cardiovascular problems, and can worsen nightly sleep, sapping energy during the day.

While there are more than 100 different forms of arthritis and related rheumatic diseases, arthritis usually includes inflammation of joints. A joint is the place where two bones meet, and arthritis can affect joints in many parts of the body: knees, hips, back, hands, elbows, fingers, ankles. Arthritis can occur due to many different reasons, but often, the affected joint becomes inflamed, and the physical components of the joint deteriorate. Bone can rub against bone with each movement, causing terrible pain.

While many people with arthritis do not show visible signs of their disease on their bodies (although it should be visible in X-rays and other tests), some people experience deformity of joints after a period of time, deformity that usually is permanent. Other people's arthritis pain may be apparent in the way they move, or in how they restrict their activities.

## Osteoarthritis and Rheumatoid Arthritis

The most common form of arthritis is *osteoarthritis,* which affects more than 20 million Americans. People tend to develop osteoarthritis, also known as OA, as they age, when their joints start to break down because they have been used repeatedly over many years of activity. Injuries to the joint and excess pressure on weight-bearing joints like the hip and knee, such as that caused by being overweight, also can lead to the development of osteoarthritis, even at a relatively young age.

In osteoarthritis, a smooth, rubbery substance in the joints called *cartilage* breaks down. Cartilage allows the bones in the joint to move properly. When cartilage breaks down, bones may rub against each other, causing pain. Loose bits of cartilage may float around in the joint, and knobby growths called *bone spurs* may form on the bones, leading to more pain.

Each joint is enclosed by the *joint capsule,* or space where the bones, *tendons* (thick, cord-like tissues that connect muscles to the bones), *ligaments* (tough tissue cords that connect the bones to each other and help them move) and sometimes, *bursae* (fluid-filled sacs that cushion the joint) meet. A thin membrane called the *synovium* lines the joint capsule. The synovium excretes a slippery liquid called *synovial fluid* that helps lubricate the joint.

In osteoarthritis, the synovium can deteriorate and the synovial fluid may decrease. This breakdown can make it harder for the bones in the joint to move properly, causing stiffness and more discomfort.

*Rheumatoid arthritis* is another common form of arthritis that can be complicated to diagnose and treat. About two million Americans have rheumatoid arthritis. RA, as it is sometimes called, is an *autoimmune disease,* or a disease where the body's immune system malfunctions. There are a number of autoimmune diseases that have chronic pain as a major symptom.

The body's disease-fighting cells secrete proteins called *antibodies.* Antibodies normally attack causes of disease that may enter the body, such as bacteria or viruses. In autoimmune diseases like RA, antibodies attack the body instead, and in these cases they are called *autoantibodies.* In the case of rheumatoid arthritis, these autoantibodies attack the joints and destroy the synovium, or joint lining, leading to inflammation, severe pain, stiffness and immobility. In RA, other organs of the body also may be affected in some cases.

## Fibromyalgia

*Fibromyalgia* is a common arthritis-related disease marked by chronic, widespread muscle pain and fatigue. About 3.7 million Americans, mostly women, are believed to have fibromyalgia at this time, although it is difficult to estimate how many people may have the disease but are undiagnosed. The numbers may be much higher.

As we learned when discussing substance P, people with fibromyalgia experience great sensitivity to pain and feel pain and tenderness throughout their body. Some particularly tender regions, known as *tender points,* usually are located near joints, which is a chief reason people with fibromyalgia sometimes are misdiagnosed with arthritis or tendinitis. People with fibromyalgia often experience other symptoms, including difficulty sleeping, anxiety, stomach distress, changes in mood, jaw pain, headaches, irritable bowel syndrome and bladder spasms. All of these problems can worsen the person's pain.

## Bursitis, Tendinitis and Similar Diseases

Bursitis, tendinitis and similar diseases known as *soft-tissue rheumatic syndromes*, affect different tissues within your joints. These conditions can be extremely painful and can reoccur often. These conditions usually don't cause permanent damage, but they can affect your daily life

Bursitis is an inflammation of the bursa, a small sac located inside the joint between bone and muscle, skin or tendon. Bursae (the plural of bursa) allow these structures to move smoothly. When injury, excessive use (such as from exercise or physical activity) or even calcium deposits cause the bursae to become inflamed, the result is severe pain and, sometimes, difficulty moving the affected joint. Pain usually lasts for only a few days to a few weeks, but it can flare again and again.

Tendinitis is an inflammation of a tendon, a thick cord that attaches muscles to bones and allows proper movement of joints. Common types of tendinitis include *rotator cuff* tendinitis (inflammation of the joints connecting the parts of the shoulder), Achilles tendinitis (inflammation of the Achilles tendon, which is located at the back of the ankle) and DeQuervain's tendinitis (inflammation of the tendons in the thumb).

There are also many common, painful disorders similar to bursitis and tendinitis, including *carpal tunnel syndrome*. A very painful and often debilitating disorder, carpal tunnel syndrome is caused by pressure on the median nerve in the wrists, which produces pain, numbness, swelling, weakness and thumb mobility problems. Sometimes, both wrists are affected.

Causes of carpal tunnel syndrome include repetitive use, such as in typing long hours at a computer keyboard, something millions of Americans do each day. Other diseases, such as thyroid gland conditions, diabetes, infection, rheumatoid arthritis or other types of inflammatory arthritis, also can lead to carpal tunnel syndrome. A small percentage of people with carpal tunnel syndrome require surgery to correct the problem and restore normal hand ability. Normally, identifying the cause and using anti-inflammatory medications will ease their painful symptoms.

The type of nerve compression found in carpal tunnel syndrome also can occur in the ankles, a condition called *tarsal tunnel syndrome*. Tarsal tunnel syndrome causes painful, burning sensations in the foot, the sole of the foot or the toes.

Another painful condition affecting the soft tissues in the joints is lateral epicondylitis, commonly known as *tennis elbow*. While you don't have to play tennis to have tennis elbow, the condition is common among people who play various sports. Any repetitive use of the wrists or clenching of the hands may cause tennis elbow. It's an inflammation of the *epicondyle,* or the area of the bone where the muscles are attached to the elbow.

Tennis elbow is a painful condition that involves an aching, persistent pain from the outside of the elbow down the forearm. Basic activities, including moving the fingers, lifting an object with the hand and wrist, turning a doorknob or opening a jar, can become painful and difficult.

When the inside of the elbow is affected, this is called medial epicondylitis, or *golfer's elbow.* Overusing the muscles used for clenching your fingers can cause golfer's elbow, which includes pain in the inner part of the elbow or pain in the fingers or wrists when bending them.

Other soft tissues can become inflamed or pressured from excessive use, causing pain, swelling and other symptoms. One such condition – called stenosing tenosynovitis or *trigger finger* – stems from a thickening of the lining around the tendons in the fingers, causing the finger to lock in a painful, bent position and then to snap open suddenly. Trigger finger can cause tenderness, swelling or small bumps in the palm, and aching pain in the middle joint of the affected finger.

Similarly, the thick, fibrous tissue stretching across the sole of your foot, from the heel to the toes, can become inflamed, a condition called *plantar fasciitis.* Plantar fasciitis, which can result from running, excessive standing, being overweight or even having "flat feet" or heel spurs, can cause pain in the sole during walking.

## Other Forms of Chronic Pain

There are many other forms of arthritis and arthritis-related diseases that involve pain that is either chronic or recurring.

- **Gout.** Gout develops due to an accumulation of a substance known as *uric acid* in the body. Gout can occur either because there is too much uric acid produced (such as from eating foods rich in *purines,* nutrients whose end-product is uric acid) or because the kidneys don't eliminate the uric acid properly, causing it to build up, crystallize and settle in joints. The primary joints affected by this crystalline build-up are those of the hands and feet. An attack of gout can be horribly painful as the build-up presses against sensitive parts of the joint and can cause inflammation.

- **Ankylosing Spondylitis.** Ankylosing spondylitis or AS is one of a group of arthritis-related diseases that primarily affect the joints of the spine. In ankylosing spondylitis, these joints can become inflamed, and eventually, the tissues supporting the spine can stiffen. The person's spine can become rigid, leading to stiffness, pain and even difficulty breathing.

- **Lupus.** Lupus or systemic lupus erythematosus (SLE) is another autoimmune disease that leads not only to joint swelling and pain but also skin rashes, internal organ damage and other serious problems. Lupus, like rheumatoid arthritis, occurs when the body's immune system, which should defend against disease-causing bacteria and viruses, turns on the body's tissues instead.

- **Back Pain.** There are many ailments that fall under the umbrella of back pain, a prevalent health problem in America today. There are many different possible causes for back pain. People may experience osteoarthritis in their back, causing pain and stiffness. Back pain also can be the result of muscle injuries or spasms, strains to the discs cushioning the spine's joints (known as *vertebrae*), compressed nerves or other problems. For example, *sciatica* is a common cause of lower back pain or even pain in the buttocks (your rear end). It's caused when the sciatic nerve, which runs from your spinal cord down your legs to your feet, is pressured or irritated. Back pain can be very intense and debilitating, or nagging and mild. In many cases, back pain recurs often.

There are many other painful forms of arthritis and related conditions, some of which you may have experienced. There are also other types of chronic pain not associated with joints or bones. Many people suffer from chronic headaches, including debilitating migraine headaches, and many people also experience terrible chronic pain related to nerve problems. No matter what the source of your pain, many of the strategies outlined in this book may help you find relief. Whether you have osteoarthritis, fibromyalgia, bursitis, nerve pain or a herniated disc in your back, your pain is real. Your pain affects your well-being and happiness. Your pain interferes with your ability to live your life normally.

That's why it is so important for you to communicate your pain to your doctor and find the appropriate treatments for your pain. Communicating what is wrong is the all-important first step in finding a solution. Yet, in some cases, this step can be the most difficult. Sometimes it's hard to describe just how and where it hurts. In this chapter, we'll show you some ways to do this effectively.

## Are All Pains Equal?

Obviously, all pains are not created equal. Pain comes in various levels of intensity due to personal situation, different causes of the pain and other reasons. Although two people may have the same disease or condition, their pain may be different, and the way they perceive and react to their pain may also differ.

Pain comes in different forms: aches, burns, stings, throbs, tingles, stabs, and on and on. The pain from stubbing your toe on the file cabinet in the office will feel very different from the pain of stepping on a nail when you're barefoot at the beach. More severe pain will elicit a much stronger chemical response from the brain: You will feel the pain faster and more intensely.

Pain can ebb and flow. If your pain chronic rather than acute, the repeated pain messages sent to the brain might affect your brain's response. Your pain may seem worse at certain times than others. A knee with arthritis may feel worse after you have been walking around the mall, for example. Your physical makeup, background, emotional state, the pain you have experienced in the past and other personal factors affect how you sense pain and react to it.

# CHILDREN AND PAIN

Many children also have chronic conditions that cause serious pain. There are more than 300,000 children with some form of juvenile arthritis or a related disease. These young people grapple with pain, fatigue, stiffness and other symptoms. Unfortunately, there are still few scientific studies on pain management in children. Many children with chronic pain conditions such as juvenile arthritis receive medications similar to those used by adults. The challenges for doctors and parents of children with chronic pain include properly assessing the intensity of the child's pain (special tests are often administered) and finding the correct dosage of drugs.

The Arthritis Foundation has many resources for children with chronic pain and their families, including:

- **Kids Get Arthritis Too,** a bimonthly newsletter published by the Arthritis Foundation with information on new research, solutions to common problems and suggestions for adapting daily activities
- **Raising a Child With Arthritis: A Parent's Guide,** a comprehensive book on juvenile arthritis and how to address pain, fatigue, emotional issues and more, including helpful exercises and relaxation strategies
- The **American Juvenile Arthritis Organization (AJAO)**, a national organization that conducts advocacy, holds periodic meetings for families and offers information to those affected by juvenile arthritis
- Other brochures and Web-based information on treatments for children with arthritis, physician referral lists, and coping and pain-management strategies

For more information, call (800) 283-7800 or log on to www.arthritis.org.

---

Let's say you and your friend are going to the church blood drive to donate blood. You have never donated blood before, and you have some anxiety and fear about the process. When the technician inserts the large needle into the vein in your arm to draw the blood, you might find the insertion shocking and painful. It may even make you feel uncomfortable and nervous. But your friend, who has donated blood many times before and has no anxiety about the process, only "feels" a slight sting. The action is the same, but the person's unique makeup creates different sensations.

It's important for you to find ways to communicate the intensity and the nature of your pain with your doctor. Doctors have many tools to help you describe and identify your pain. They might ask you to rate your pain or describe it in detail through a series of tests (see p. 33).

Your medical examination will include a medical history, during which your doctor or a nurse will ask you all sorts of questions about your past medical problems and what medications you may have taken. The medical history also is likely to include various tests, if necessary, to determine the nature of your problem and the underlying cause of your pain. Again, by pinpointing the cause of your pain, your doctor will be able to prescribe the right medications and suggest the appropriate measures to address your pain.

In some cases, medical tests and questions may not immediately reveal the cause of your pain or an appropriate course of action. It's important for you to stay optimistic! While you may have to learn to deal with certain amounts of pain in your life, pain should not become so overwhelming that you have to stay in bed for a week or not be able to walk to the mailbox. You and your doctor should continue to try various methods for treating your pain.

If necessary, you may have to consult a specialist, a doctor with additional training in certain medical fields. If you have arthritis that is causing more than mild, occasional pain and stiffness, you might consult a rheumatologist, a doctor who has years of additional training in treating arthritis and related rheumatic diseases (such as those described earlier in this chapter). Or, your pain may become so intense that you require surgical treatment from an *orthopaedic surgeon,* a doctor who specializes in surgery of the bones and joints.

If you have chronic, debilitating pain and need special, ongoing treatment for that pain, you might consult an *anesthesiologist* who specializes in pain medicine. These doctors, rather than just performing anesthesia for surgery (which numbs you or makes you sleep while the operation is happening), can help treat your pain and administer various pain treatments that we will discuss in this book. These doctors may also be known as pain specialists or pain doctors.

## Finding Ways to Fight Pain

Pain, as we said earlier, is a unique experience for each person. Some people may have mild chronic pain that only becomes bothersome on an occasional basis. Other people may have intense pain that interferes with their ability to work and live a normal life.

It's up to you to determine what is tolerable for you. Together with your doctor, you should be able to find some strategies that relieve your pain. You should not have to "grin and bear it" when there are many treatments that can control pain.

Some people worry about the *side effects* of painkilling drugs or other drugs. These effects, which can range from stomach disorders to constipation to grogginess, are a real concern for many people. Some drugs can have dangerous or life-threatening side effects, so it's important for you to let your doctor know immediately if one of these effects occurs.

Your doctor should be able to work with

you to find the right drugs, or combination of drugs if necessary, and the proper dosage of the drug to keep you from having excessive side effects. But if side effects are becoming a health hazard of their own, let your doctor know. You may have to switch drugs, lower the dosage you take, or try other methods of relieving your pain. Later, we will outline some ways to deal with side effects of common drugs.

Not all pain-control strategies involve drugs or other medical treatments. There are many other ways to relieve pain. We will learn about many of these methods in this book. Exercise, diet, alternative therapies like *acupuncture* or *herbal supplements*, movement techniques like *yoga, tai chi* or the *Alexander Technique* also can help you alleviate your pain. Relaxation techniques can reduce your stress, easing pain by relaxing tense muscles. Drugs, surgery and medical devices may help you fight pain in most cases, but these other therapies can accentuate medical treatments and be very effective.

One of the most powerful weapons you have in the battle against pain is your mind. Your brain is the center of pain perception, as well as the center of emotions that govern how you respond to pain. Your brain also contains great power to deal with pain and even lessen pain. In this book, you will learn strategies to harness your mind's power to fight pain, including *guided imagery* and *meditation*. With these methods and more, you may be able to close that pain gate or, at least, narrow it so pain does not take over your life.

In the next chapter, we will look at how your doctor will diagnose the cause of your pain and take the first steps in recommending treatments.

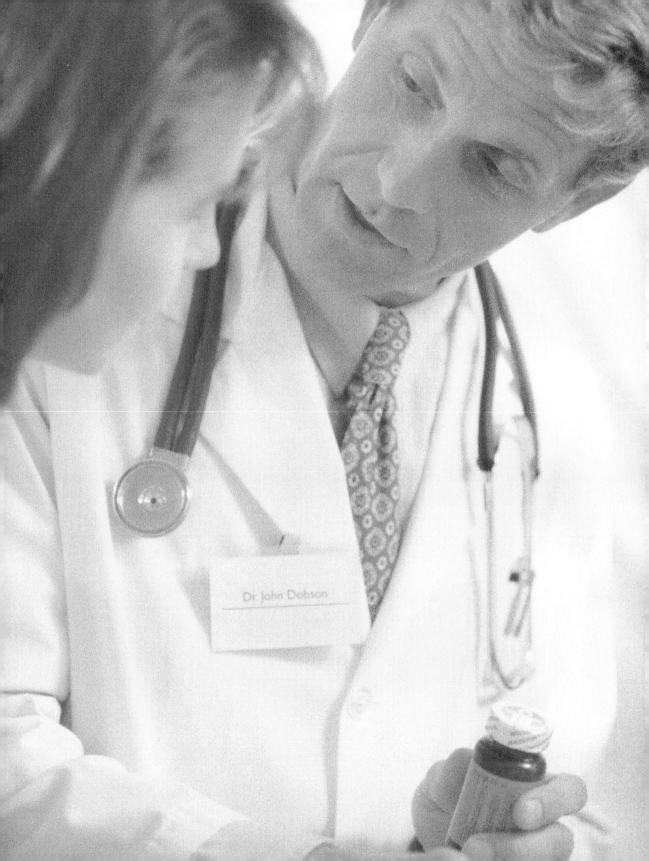

# What's Causing
# Your Pain?

2

# CHAPTER 2: WHAT'S CAUSING YOUR PAIN?

When you have serious, chronic pain that doesn't go away with over-the-counter treatments or rest, your first action should be to pick up the phone and make an appointment with your doctor. Your second action should be – in partnership with your doctor – doing what it takes to find the cause of your pain. Only when you know what causes your pain can you move to the third step: creating a comprehensive pain-management plan that works.

Other than its origins and its duration, how does chronic pain differ from acute pain? Chronic pain – such as the pain of arthritis, fibromyalgia, nerve damage, spinal cord injuries, or even serious diseases such as cancer – involves a slightly different process than acute pain.

In acute pain, such as that from a short-term stomach illness, a burn or injury, is a sudden shock to the body. Nerves specializing in sensing pain release chemicals that send alarm-like pain messages up the spinal cord and to the brain. The brain feels as if the body is in danger, so it responds with a sudden flare of pain. In some cases, powerful drugs, such as opioids like codeine, can be used on a short-term basis to relieve severe pain of short duration.

Chronic pain may be more complex to treat. Because the problems causing the pain are present over a long period of time, and probably worsen over time, pain-sensitive nerves can become even more sensitive to the stimulus. Some researchers believe that repeated stimulation might cause these nerves to send continuous pain signals to the brain even when the pain-causing condition has been treated or resolved.

So treating chronic pain can be difficult for doctors and patients alike. Many people do not like the prospect of taking painkilling drugs on a regular, long-term basis. However, there are new types of drugs and other treatments that may lessen chronic pain effectively.

## FINDING PAIN'S CAUSE

As we learned in Chapter One, you and your doctor are not just treating the pain. You are searching for the disease or problem that is causing the pain. Treatments may address the disease – such as osteoarthritis, rheumatoid arthritis, fibromyalgia or gout, for example – that has pain as one of its symptoms.

If you have rheumatoid arthritis, for example, your doctor might prescribe a *corticosteroid* medication such as prednisone, or a slow-acting *disease-modifying antirheumatic drug*, such as methotrexate, to address the inflammation or the immune system malfunction that is causing your joints to swell and hurt. In some cases, you might need additional treatments, both medical and alternative, to relieve the pain itself.

Before you can begin to discuss treating your pain, you and your doctor must pinpoint pain's cause. You have to find an effective way of communicating the nature and intensity of your pain to your doctor and other members of the health-care team, such as *nurses* or *physician assistants*. It's vital that you make the most of the short time you may have to talk to your doctor about your pain and related symptoms so that you can find an effective treatment for your pain as soon as possible.

In this chapter, we will discuss techniques your doctor may use to diagnose the cause of your pain, and further explain the main causes of chronic pain that you may be experiencing. We also will show you ways to communicate more effectively and efficiently with your doctor and his staff.

## Diagnosis: Tests and Questions

Diagnosis is the first and most important step in pain treatment. The word "diagnosis" comes from the Greek word meaning "to distinguish," and the process of diagnosis involves distinguishing your problem based on an examination of all the facts about your health problem. Like a detective, your doctor and members of his staff will ask you various questions and perform tests, if necessary, to gather information about you and your health.

During your first appointment, your doctor probably will take the following steps to form a diagnosis:

- Take a *medical history*, asking you about your past health problems, medical procedures or injuries, and health problems that your close family members may have had

- Discuss all the medications and other therapies you currently use (not only for pain, but for other health problems as well)

- Conduct a through physical examination

- Use some type of pain assessment test, such as a pain scale or questionnaire, or just talk to you about your pain

- Test blood, urine or other bodily fluids

- In some instances, conduct tests such as X-rays, magnetic resonance imaging tests (MRI), computerized axial tomography (CAT or CT) scans, dual X-ray absorptiometry (DEXA) scans and others to examine bones and soft tissues

These techniques and tests will help your doctor determine the probable cause of your pain as well as joint damage or other problems that may already have occurred in the body. These facts will help your doctor decide what steps to take to treat your pain.

Communicating your pain is the most important first step in treatment. Your doctor might talk to you or give you tests designed to gather and qualify data about your pain. Answer these questions as truthfully as possible. Try not to exaggerate or downplay any problems you have. If possible, before your appointment with your doctor, write down a basic description of your problems and a timeline of when and how they occurred. Also have a brief medical history ready for your doctor if you have not discussed this with your doctor before. See p. 30 for more information about your medical history.

## What If You Don't Have a Doctor?

You may be in pain – but what if you don't know whom to call for help?

Not everyone has an established relationship with a doctor or a *primary-care physician* (usually an internist or family physician). There are many reasons why you may not have a doctor to turn to. You may have changed insurance coverage and your physician does not accept your new plan. You may not have insurance coverage at this time due to job change or your personal situation. You may have relocated to a new residence and don't know the doctors in your new neighborhood. Your previous doctor may have retired. Or, until now, you never felt the need to have a doctor. But now you do. What do you do?

Whether or not a person has a chronic illness or any illness at all, it's important to have some kind of ongoing, regular care from a *health-care professional.* This professional will monitor your overall health and address problems as needed. When you feel sick or become injured, you will be able to turn to a professional who understands your particular situation and past medical problems.

If you are experiencing chronic pain, it's very important to have a regular relationship with a doctor. It's likely that you will need ongoing care for your health problem and periodic office visits to monitor treatment and progress. Here are a few important questions (and answers) for you to ponder as you begin your search.

**What kind of doctor am I looking for?** This is really up to you. You may wish to begin seeing a primary-care physician, internist or family physician, all terms for doctors who diagnose and treat a wide variety of health problems. This doctor may be allopathic, known as a *medical doctor* or "MD," or he or she may be an *osteopathic doctor* or "DO." An MD is a doctor whose graduate medical degree conformed to traditional medical philosophy, while a DO's philosophy of medicine may be slightly different. Osteopaths follow a medical philosophy based on the idea that most illness is linked to problems in the musculoskeletal system, such as when bones are not in their proper position. However, their training is very similar to that of allopathic doctors, and their qualifications to treat disease and pain are the same. Both osteopaths and medical doctors can prescribe drugs and perform surgery if necessary.

Depending on your situation, insurance coverage, age or even your gender, you may wish to see a *specialist* on a regular basis. A specialist is a doctor who completed years of specialized study in a particular medical field. While these doctors may be MDs or DOs, they focus on certain illnesses or fields of medicine. Specialists you might see regularly include a gynecologist (specializing in women's health care), a rheumatologist (specializing in arthritis and rheumatic diseases), a cardiologist (specializing in heart diseases) or even a pain specialist. Your primary-care physician – the "regular doctor" that guides your normal health care – can refer you to a specialist if necessary.

**Where do I find names of doctors and other health-care professionals?** There are many ways to choose a doctor. Your insurance coverage (if you have it) will narrow your search. If you have medical insurance, you probably will wish to choose a doctor whose services are covered by your policy. Some policies allow you to choose from a list of physicians (including specialists) that are covered. You would have to pay a set fee for the medical visit, or a *copayment*. Other policies allow you to use a doctor who is not included on this list, but will still pay for a percentage of the fees. If you do not have an insurance policy or you have one that does not cover regular office visits to a doctor, you will have to pay for the services yourself.

*Referrals* are recommendations from friends, family, coworkers or medical professionals. Ask people you know and trust to refer you to their doctor, and compare this list to your insurance policy's list of covered doctors. If you find some professionals who match both lists, call their offices and see if you can make an appointment for an *initial consultation*. You may wish to talk to the doctor before you commit to ongoing care to see if he or she is right for you.

The local Yellow Pages phone directory also will have a listing of doctors, divided by specialty and office locations. You can also search the Internet for medical associations that list their members by geographical location. For example, organizations such as the American College of Rheumatology, the American Academy of Orthopaedic Surgeons, the American

Society of Anesthesiologists and the American Association of Family Physicians have listings of their member specialists, including contact information. Your local chapter of the Arthritis Foundation can also provide a list of arthritis specialists in your area; contact the Arthritis Foundation at (800) 283-7800 or www.arthritis.org to find the nearest office. Again, compare these lists to the doctors listed in your insurance policy directory.

**What factors should influence my choice of doctor?** A number of factors will help you decide which doctors are good candidates to become *your* doctor. Whether or not the doctors accept your insurance policy or Medicare will be a major deciding factor. You will have to pay more if a doctor's service is not covered by your insurance. In addition, you may wish to consider the following:

- The location of the doctor's office or offices: Is it convenient?
- The size of the staff in the office: Do they have enough staff to handle the patient load?
- The personality of the doctor and/or his staff: Do they make you feel comfortable? Are they courteous? Do they listen and make eye contact with you?
- Other facts about the doctor: Is the doctor's gender or age important to you? Can you relate to the doctor and discuss your problems?
- The responsiveness of the doctor and his staff: When you call to make an appointment, request a prescription or ask a ques-

tion, do they respond in a timely manner? Can you leave messages easily?

- The size of the doctor's practice: Does the office seem too large or impersonal for you? Or is it too small, creating a backlog of patients and excessive waiting time?
- The doctor's experience and training: Do you feel confident in his ability? Is the doctor "board-certified"? What credentials does he have?
- The time your doctor usually spends with a patient: Do you feel that he offers you enough time to discuss your problems?
- The hospital your doctor uses: Is it conveniently located should you need to be admitted to the hospital? Do you feel comfortable using this hospital in case you need surgery or hospital services?
- The experiences of other patients: Do other people who use this doctor speak well of him, his office, his staff and his services?

When you narrow your choices, you may wish to ask the doctor or his staff the following important questions:

- Does this doctor or practice accept new patients at this time?
- What insurance policies are accepted and how are payments handled?
- Will this doctor handle pre-certification for medical procedures?
- What are the days of the week and hours that the office is open for appointments?
- Typically, how much advance notice is needed to make appointments?

- How much advance notice is needed to cancel an appointment?
- On average, how long does the doctor spend with each patient? What about support staff?
- If I have an emergency, how quickly can I arrange an appointment?
- How are emergencies that require hospitalization handled by the doctor?
- What can I do if I have a medical problem after hours or when the doctor is on vacation?

**Remember:** Your choice of doctor is important. If you are not satisfied, you can always seek the services of another doctor. Speak frankly to your doctor about your needs and concerns. Chances are, your doctor wishes to make you feel well treated as well as to treat your health problems.

## Pain Centers and Pain Clinics

Your primary-care doctor will diagnose the cause of your pain and begin the treatment process. If you and your doctor don't find adequate pain relief from the treatments your doctor suggests, he can, if necessary, refer you to a pain specialist. These doctors may have various medical backgrounds, but many are anesthesiologists with additional pain-management training. You may associate anesthesiologists with surgery, and these doctors do often work in surgical settings to anesthetize the patient during the procedure (so he or she doesn't feel the horrible pain of the operation). Some anesthesiologists specialize in treating ongoing pain and offer helpful treatments and long-term pain-management techniques.

Pain specialists may have their own medical practices, or they may work in hospitals or in special institutions that focus only on pain treatment. These special facilities are called *pain centers* or *pain clinics*. A pain center is an institution where doctors of various specialties work together to address a wide variety of chronic pain problems. Each doctor has a different area of expertise, and all can consult together on patients in pain. In addition, the pain center probably has nurses, physician assistants, physical therapists, occupational therapists and, perhaps, psychologists on staff to help you adapt to your pain or deal with the emotional impact of chronic pain.

Pain centers, which often are associated with universities, medical schools or large hospital complexes, also might have health-professionals from other disciplines on staff to advise you about your overall health and fitness. These professionals might include counselors, social workers, dietitians or nutritionists, or even a pastor. Pain affects your whole life, including your job and your personal relationships. These professionals may help you adjust to your chronic pain, or help you find ways to make positive improvements (such as to lose excess weight) to your health to increase pain relief.

A pain clinic typically is a smaller institution, a place where one or maybe a few doctors who specialize in pain treatment consult with and treat chronic pain patients. These doctors can help diagnose the cause of your pain, prescribe treatments and monitor your ongoing process. They may not be able to provide the comprehensive approach of a pain

center, but their care may be adequate to addressing your pain-management needs.

Some pain centers offer an intensive, inpatient treatment that may last up to four weeks. These inpatient treatments are more expensive than outpatient pain-management programs, and would not be for everyone. Enrolling in this type of treatment also would require your spending a significant amount of time away from work and family. Again, it may not be possible for everyone. Insurance coverage for such treatment varies greatly, so you should explore your policy's coverage before making any commitment to a treatment program.

During the period when you are a patient in the pain center, you would receive intense, personal evaluation and monitoring. Not only would you undergo drug treatments, but you also would learn methods, both physical and emotional, for managing your pain. Staff members could observe you around the clock to pinpoint behavior patterns that might worsen your pain, and help you address these behaviors. Outpatient programs cost less and involve less concentrated attention.

When you go to a pain center or pain clinic, the pain specialist probably will repeat some of the basic testing that your primary-care doctor conducted. You can expect to have a physical examination, perhaps undergo some diagnostic tests (like X-rays) and discuss your medical history. These steps allow the doctor to confirm your diagnosis and suggest possible treatment.

Then, the doctor will discuss the pros and cons of the available treatments. Once you decide together how to proceed, your treatment begins. If you don't find adequate relief, your doctor will try other treatments to continue the search for a solution.

If you don't have a pain center or pain clinic in your area, it's very likely that your primary-care doctor can administer the pain-relief methods described in this chapter, or refer you to a specialist who can. If necessary, you may have to travel some distance to see a pain specialist. Make arrangements with a friend or family member to accompany you to these sessions if possible. Be sure to review your insurance policy to see if these more advanced pain-relief methods are covered. Some policies may only cover standard drug treatments. Pre-certification of diagnostic and treatment procedures may be necessary.

What happens if you don't find a medical treatment that relieves your pain? Your pain specialist may be able to help you learn how to adapt to your new situation, difficult as it may be. This process, called *pain rehabilitation,* means learning ways to modify your activities, use non-medical techniques to relax or cope with the stress of chronic pain, find a support network of friends or family members to help you handle daily tasks, and try various non-drug or even alternative pain-relief techniques to help you manage your pain.

The first step in any doctor's or health-care professional's treatment will be to get some background information on you, your painful condition and your general health state. To begin, he or she will probably take a medical history.

## What Is Your Medical History?

A medical history is the story of your health. This story includes chapters about illnesses, injuries or health problems you have had in the past; your record of vaccinations; allergies; any health conditions or medical problems your close family members have had; and medications or treatments you have used, and any side effects they may have caused. These pieces of information come together to a form your health profile, often revealing where you may be at risk for developing certain diseases or problems. Also, your medical history suggests what treatments may or may not be effective for you.

When you make your first appointment with a new doctor, the staff will ask you to fill out some forms about your medical history, current state of health, insurance coverage and other important facts. Your doctor (or a nurse or physician assistant) will go over your medical history face to face during your consultation. They will keep a record of this information so they can refer to it on future visits.

However, it may be helpful for you to write down your own medical history before you go to your appointment. By doing this, you will be able to remember problems you may have had long ago, and you will have the opportunity to contact relatives if you have questions about diseases that may be common in your family.

A few days before your appointment, spend an hour or so writing down what medical problems you have had during your lifetime. Include major injuries or illnesses, such as a car accident, recurring episodes of back pain, a broken bone that required medical care, pneumonia or chickenpox. List what immunizations you have had, and check past medical records for this information if you have them. Try to recall if you have ever had any unusual test results in your blood, urine, blood pressure, heartbeat or reflexes. Have you ever been told that you have high blood pressure? Have you gained or lost a great deal of weight in the past? Have you had major surgery for any reason?

In addition, what sort of examinations or tests have you had in the past – such as a blood test, mammogram, Pap smear, prostate exam or colonoscopy – and what were the results? You or your doctor can request important test results from your past doctors if necessary. It's important to note if you or your parents, grandparents or siblings ever had any major illnesses or health problems, including:

- Diabetes
- Stroke
- Heart attack or heart problems
- Cancer
- Arthritis or a related disease
- Osteoporosis
- Gastrointestinal diseases
- Alcoholism or drug abuse
- High blood pressure
- Depression
- Other major health problems

If your parents or grandparents had some diseases or health problems, you may be more at risk for developing them. This doesn't mean that you are certain to get this illness – it just means that you should be aware of the warning signs, and make lifestyle changes if necessary. Your doctor and his staff will ask follow-up questions if they need to know more about your medical past. These facts all blend together to create your health profile. Using this profile, your doctor will be able to address any problems and monitor your ongoing health care.

You can request a copy of your medical history to keep at home. It may be helpful for you to have this information for visits to other doctors or specialists, or in case you are admitted to the hospital in an emergency. It may be good to have this data on hand for you and your family.

## Talking to Your Doctor About Pain

Once you go over your medical history, members of your doctor's staff will probably perform a few basic tests to assess your current physical condition. The nurse may weigh you; take your blood pressure, pulse and temperature; perform a "finger-prick" blood test to assess your iron level or other basic data; and ask you to urinate in a small cup to test your urine.

Don't be frustrated by a battery of tests: They're necessary for your doctor to get a clearer picture of your situation. Even though these tests may not specifically relate to your pain, they will help your doctor assess your overall health. Your health may have an impact on your pain whether you realize it or not. For example, if you are overweight for your height and age, the excess pounds may be putting too much stress on your hips and knees. If you have arthritis in your hips or knees, this might make the pain worse.

When you have completed some tests, your doctor or a member of his support staff probably will ask you some questions about your pain and related symptoms. They'll want to know what prompted you to make your doctor's appointment. It's important to communicate your problems effectively to the doctor because he may not have a great deal of time to spend with you. So make the most of that time! If you prepare a bit before your appointment, you'll be one step ahead in the process.

As we suggested you do with your medical history, sit down for a little while before your appointment to think about your symptoms. Create a summary of your condition by writing informal notes about what you are feeling. Ask yourself the following questions to help you form your summary:

- **How does the pain feel?** Try to find words that describe the actual sensation, such as burning, aching, tingling, stinging, etc.
- **Where does the pain occur in the body?** Be as specific as possible. For instance, does your leg hurt? At the thigh, the hip, the knee or the ankle?
- **When does pain occur?** Does pain worsen at certain times of day, such as late afternoon after you have been sitting at your desk all day, or in connection with certain activities, such as after you exercise?
- **Do you experience other symptoms on a regular basis?** Note anything that seems

unusual, such as stomach pain, nausea, fatigue, inability to fall asleep, headaches, pain with sexual activity, etc. Do these symptoms seem to occur in connection with your pain?
- **How long have you been experiencing this pain?** Did it start suddenly, or did you notice it gradually?
- **How intense is the pain?** Is it mild but annoying? Or is it so intense at times that you cannot function, sleep, move your joint, have sex, or perform other daily, necessary activities? Pain intensity may be difficult to describe to your doctor. Your doctor can offer you some helpful mechanisms for doing so.

## How to Describe Pain

Pain is a personal experience that is very difficult to describe to others. Two people with very similar disease situations may perceive their pain differently. Many factors may affect how you perceive and react to pain: personal history, personality, cultural makeup, gender, age and others.

Arthritis pain is also very subjective. Arthritis can involve many different symptoms, affect different joints and organs, and manifest distinctly from one person to the next. One standard of arthritis pain is that it is chronic. However, each person may find that the pain worsens at some times and lessens at others.

It's important for you to figure out the patterns in your pain and what factors may trigger or alleviate your pain, and to communicate this information to your doctor. To help understand your pain, your doctor may use various tools to help him "rank" or qualify that pain. These tools include:

- **Pain scales,** which are charts designed to help you rank the intensity of your pain. For example, you might rank the pain you experience on a scale of 1 to 10, where 1 is feeling perfectly well and 10 is the worst pain imaginable. Your pain might vary in intensity depending on certain factors, and this scale would help you explain to your doctor the variance between times when your pain is tolerable and times when your pain flares or gets suddenly worse.
- **Pain questionnaires,** which are a series of questions about your pain, where it is located, what words or comparisons you can use to describe it, what makes it worse, and other factors. For example, you might feel "burning" in your left hip that gets worse after you have been on your feet all day at work, or a "dull ache" and "stiffness" in your knees that is worst in the morning and gets better

after your shower. There are many different types of pain questionnaires, but these tools allow you to explain important facts about your pain to your doctor so he can evaluate the nature of your problem. A complete example of an actual pain questionnaire used by pain specialists is included at the end of this chapter.

- **Pain diaries or journals** are another way for you to track your pain over a period of time. Your doctor might ask you to keep a diary or journal for several days or weeks before your next appointment, noting when pain occurs, what parts of the body are affected by pain, the nature or intensity of the pain, and other important points. Pain diaries allow your doctor to note patterns in your pain, what factors may cause pain flares, what other symptoms may accompany your pain, and what treatments may have worked or not worked to alleviate your pain.

All of the tools your doctor uses to assess your pain, and the information they provide, help your doctor diagnose the cause of the pain and determine treatment options. Different treatments might work better than others depending on the cause of your pain, your lifestyle, what treatments have worked in the past, and other factors.

## DIAGNOSIS: PHYSICAL EXAMS AND MEDICAL TESTS

During the physical examination, your doctor may look at the joint or joints where your pain occurs, and may ask you to move the

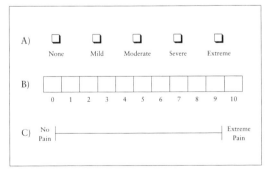

QUALIFYING PAIN: Examples of various pain scales.

affected area. He may look for swelling, stiffness, redness or other obvious symptoms in and around the joint that point to the cause of your pain.

Your doctor also may check other parts of your body, such as the skin, eyes or mouth, to determine if you have certain illnesses that affect these organs. These signs can tell your doctor that you have certain forms of arthritis, or rule these diseases out as the cause of your chronic pain. The doctor might also ask you to walk, sit or bend to observe your gait, the curvature of your spine, the height of your shoulders or other signs.

If your pain and other symptoms suggest you might have fibromyalgia, your doctor will perform a *tender point exam*. Diagnosing fibromyalgia is often imprecise and time-consuming, as medical research has not yet confirmed the true cause of fibromyalgia. However, the American College of Rheumatology (ACR), the official organization of rheumatologists that issues official medical guidelines and research studies concerning arthritis and related diseases, developed some official criteria for a diagnosis of fibromyalgia. These criteria help doctors rule out other problems and confirm a diagnosis of fibromyalgia.

People with fibromyalgia do not have swelling, pain or stiffness in joints themselves, as seen in arthritis. Instead, they have pain and, often, extreme tenderness or sensitivity in certain areas of the body. These areas are known as tender points. A person with fibromyalgia must have pain and sensitivity in at least 11 of the 18 recognized tender points. During a ten-

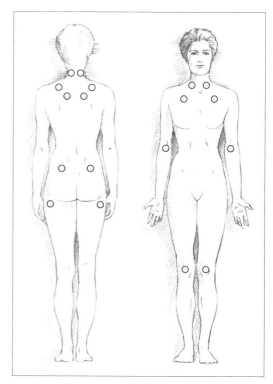

TENDER POINTS: Points of the body where fibromyalgia pain is most common

der point exam, the physician applies pressure to the 18 points and counts the number of sites where unusual pain and sensitivity occurs. The chart on this page shows the 18 recognized tender points of fibromyalgia.

In order to diagnose the cause of your chronic pain, your doctor may issue a variety of medical tests. These tests may rule out certain ailments as well as suggest them. We mentioned a few of these types of tests above, but here, we'll go into a little more detail about common tests used to diagnose arthritis and related diseases. Again, with fibromyalgia, the only reliable test at this time is the tender point exam and a verbal discussion of symptoms. But for other diseases that can cause chronic pain, body fluid and imagery tests can aid in diagnosis.

## Laboratory Tests

Your blood, urine and other fluids can hold clues to the cause of your pain. For example, if tests show that you have abnormally high or low levels of certain chemicals in your body fluids, they might suggest the existence of certain diseases. That's why it's important for your doctor to take a urine sample and/or a small blood sample.

Here is a rundown of some common tests used to diagnose arthritis and related diseases, chief causes of chronic pain:

Anti-DNA test. The anti-DNA blood test detects the presence of autoantibodies in the blood. Antibodies are substances made by the body that attach to disease-causing foreign agents like viruses or bacteria and help the body defend itself against their attack. Sometimes, antibodies behave wrongly and mistakenly attack one's own DNA (the material found in the nucleus of each human cell that serves as the basic building block of life). The presence of these autoantibodies (or antibodies-gone-wrong) is a common sign of lupus.

Anti-nuclear antibody test. Also known as an ANA test, this blood test shows the existence of antibodies that mistakenly attack the nuclei (command centers) of cells, leading to cell damage. A positive result may be evidence of an autoimmune disease. ANA tests are used in diagnosis of lupus, rheumatoid arthritis, scleroderma (an arthritis-related disease involving skin damage), polymyositis (an inflammatory disease affecting muscle) and others.

Complement test. This blood test measures the level of complement, a substance that aids the body's own immune system, our defense against disease. Complement helps antibodies do their job in fighting foreign agents, such as bacteria and viruses. When levels of complement are too low, this may indicate that the person has an autoimmune disease such as vasculitis (a term for diseases marked by inflammation of the blood vessels) or lupus.

Complete blood count test (CBC). Complete blood count testing measures various components in the blood, which can be indicators of certain types of diseases. A low number of red blood cells, a condition known as *anemia,* could indicate rheumatoid arthritis, lupus, polymyalgia rheumatica, inflammatory bowel disease or other diseases. A low count of white blood cells (which help fight disease) or platelets might indicate lupus. A high count of white blood cells might indicate an infection.

C-Reactive protein test. C-reactive protein (or CRP) is a plasma protein found in the blood. High levels of this protein are an indicator of inflammation. High levels of CRP can be seen in cases of physical trauma, burns, advanced stages of cancer, surgery and inflammatory diseases. The CRP test is used commonly in the process of diagnosing rheumatoid arthritis and other diseases marked by inflammation. Elevated levels of CRP alone is not a sure sign of any one condition, but this test can help the doctor determine a diagnosis along with other methods.

Erythrocyte sedimentation rate or "sed rate" test. A sed rate blood test measures how fast red blood cells fall to the bottom of the test tube. Substances in the blood that cause inflammation also may make red blood cells clump together. Because these heavy clumps fall faster than single red blood cells, a high "sed rate," or the rate at which red blood cells are falling, can indicate inflammation in the body. This test often is used to diagnose rheumatoid arthritis, ankylosing spondylitis, polymyalgia rheumatica and other arthritis-related diseases that have painful inflammation as a symptom.

Joint fluid exam. In a joint fluid exam, doctors withdraw fluid from the cavity of the joint, which can then be tested for the presence of certain chemicals or elements. This test can help diagnose painful diseases like gout, because uric acid crystals would be present in the joint fluid. If joint fluid tests show bacteria, it may mean that a person has *infectious arthritis*, a form of arthritis caused by a bacterial infection.

Lyme serology test. The Lyme serology blood test looks for particular antibodies that react to *Borrelia burgdorferi,* the bacteria that cause *Lyme disease*. Lyme disease, caused by a bite from an infected tick, can cause fever, muscle and joint pain, fatigue and other symptoms.

Rheumatoid factor test (also known as RA latex test). Rheumatoid factor testing reveals the presence of the rheumatoid factor autoantibody, or RF. Many people with rheumatoid arthritis produce large amounts of rheumatoid factor, so this test may indicate a diagnosis of RA. However, some people who do not have RA also test positive for this autoantibody, so the test doesn't confirm the disease without other evidence.

Tissue typing test. Tissue typing is used to confirm the presence of certain genetic markers or signs in the blood that may indicate certain diseases. If the test reveals that the person has a marker called HLA-B27, for example, it may indicate a diagnosis of ankylosing spondylitis or reactive arthritis, a disease marked by painful inflammation of the joints, eyes or urethra.

Uric acid test. In a uric acid test, levels of uric acid, a waste product produced by cells in the body, are measured. If uric acid levels are too high, it may indicate the person has gout.

Urinalysis. Urinalysis is a general testing of the urine can help to detect kidney or urinary tract infections, or other similar health problems that cause changes to your urine. High levels of certain elements, such as uric acid or protein, can aid in diagnosis of disease.

## Imaging Tests

X-rays and similar tests use radiation – often in extremely small amounts – to produce images that reveal the inside of your body. Doctors use these images to examine the joints and other structures for signs of damage that may be causing pain. In some cases, these tests are administered and reviewed by a specialist known as a *radiologist.* If you need to have a special imaging test, your doctor will refer you to a radiologist to perform the necessary procedure.

Here's a rundown of some of the most common imaging tests used in diagnosing chronic pain conditions, such as back problems, arthritis and related diseases.

X-rays. X-ray images, or *radiographs*, are created when controlled electromagnetic radiation is beamed through the part of the body being examined. X-rays are used to diagnose many diseases and injuries, from arthritis to a broken bone. Your doctor can use radiographs to see what's under your skin and muscles, and to view the bones and connective tissue that make up your joints.

An X-ray image can show problems that could be causing pain. X-rays can indicate the presence of a *tumor* (which could be cancerous or *malignant,* or non-cancerous or *benign*) or mass that may be causing pain by pressing against organs, bones or tissues. X-rays also can show fractures (or breaks) in bones. A fracture in a vertebra, one of the bones that make up the spine, might cause back pain and need to be treated. X-rays are limited some-

what in their ability to reveal some soft-tissue problems, but they can assess soft-tissue masses pressing against bones, as well as calcification (or hardening) within soft tissues that may be causing pain. In some cases, other, more precise new imaging methods may help the doctor more.

X-rays can reveal various problems associated with a chronic disease like osteoarthritis. By reviewing the type of joint damage seen on your X-ray, doctors can pinpoint the disease that is causing your pain. By looking at an X-ray of a joint affected by osteoarthritis, a doctor can see if the space between the two bones that make up the joint is too narrow and uneven due to the wear and damage OA causes to the cartilage in the joint. X-rays might also reveal bone spurs, painful outcroppings at the ends of bones. X-ray images showing inflammation in the joints of the spine might suggest ankylosing spondylitis or a similar disease.

While X-rays are very commonly used in diagnosis, X-ray technology does involve exposure to radiation. Read the short article "Are X-rays Harmful?" on page 38 to learn more about the risks and what precautions you should take.

DEXA. DEXA scans, an abbreviation for dual energy X-ray absorptiometry, are a very reliable way to diagnose osteoporosis, a disease marked by thinning bones. For this reason, many people refer to DEXA scans as "bone density tests." People with osteoporosis are at an increased risk for serious bone breaks, and

## ARE X-RAYS HARMFUL?

As X-rays beam radiation through part of your body in order to create the image that your doctor reviews, it is understandable that you would be concerned about the risk. Too much exposure to radiation could harm the body, even leading to diseases such as cancer. Most people will not have nearly enough X-rays to incur this risk.

Even so, doctors should use X-rays only when necessary, and only take enough X-rays to get the job done without putting you at too much risk for radiation's possible effects. Your doctor or his staff members will "shoot" only the area of your body that needs examination. In some cases, they will cover parts of your torso and lower body (especially where your sex organs sit) with a lead apron to shield you from excess radiation that could be harmful.

If you are a woman, it's important that you tell your doctor or his staff if you think you may be pregnant. Radiation from an X-ray could be harmful to a fetus. So speak up if you are pregnant or even if you think you are pregnant.

Some alternative health-care practitioners may administer multiple diagnostic X-rays as part of their initial treatment. This should not be necessary in most cases, and it could be dangerous. Speak up if you have concerns about excessive X-rays as part of any pain diagnosis. Your doctor may have already taken X-rays of painful areas of your body, and you could provide these images to your practitioner instead.

DEXA scans help to assess that risk. The images measure bone density to determine if your bones are becoming weaker or more porous (full of tiny holes).

Women who may be at risk for osteoporosis – those at or past menopause or those who have taken bone-thinning glucocorticoid medications for diseases like rheumatoid arthritis – are most likely to have DEXA scans to diagnose the disease.

DEXA scans use less radiation than a traditional X-ray. When you have a DEXA scan, you lie on a table while the DEXA imaging machine passes over you. It is not painful and only lasts about 15 to 20 minutes.

MRI. You've probably seen the term MRI (short for magnetic resonance imaging) often in the news, especially on the sports pages. It seems like baseball pitchers are always having

MRIs on their injured elbows and shoulders. These scans help see a much more detailed internal image of the body, so doctors can diagnose problems associated with bones as well as soft tissues.

When you have an MRI, you lie on a long, narrow table. The table moves you into a big, enclosed tube where a strong magnet passes a force through your body. The magnetic force creates a computerized image of a cross section of the area of your body your doctor needs to examine. The image is very detailed. The whole process may take up to an hour. Because of the length of the process, some people find MRI uncomfortable, particularly people who are claustrophobic or fearful of enclosed spaces. A new MRI machine called "open MRI" is less confining. Open MRI may not produce images of the same detail as traditional MRI, however, and it might not be available in some areas.

Many people with arthritis or related diseases have MRI scans to determine different pain-causing problems. Bone loss, knee injuries and other types of joint problems can be diagnosed through MRI technology.

MRI does not use radiation, so in some ways it is safer than X-rays. However, there are other potential problems with using MRI. If you have a pacemaker or other type of metal implant (such as those used in joint replacements or spine surgery) within your body, you may not be able to use MRI due to the magnetic element. Your doctor or the MRI operators should ask you if you have either of these devices, but speak up if they do not ask.

CT or CAT Scan. Computerized axial tomography, commonly called CT or CAT scans, may be used in some cases to diagnose painful conditions or injuries to bones or internal organs. CT scans are similar to X-rays, but use a computer to create a more detailed image of the internal structures of the body or a specific area. CT scans may be useful in diagnosing back or spine problems such as fractured vertebrae, or to identify tumors. CT scans and MRI can be more expensive than other types of scans, so they are often reserved for diagnosing problems that cannot be diagnosed using regular X-rays.

Bone scans, myelography and discography. Bone scans, myelograms and discograms are imaging techniques that involve injecting a special dye into the body to illuminate or highlight areas of inflammation or damage. These techniques are often used in diagnosing painful back or spinal cord problems. They may be used prior to surgery to help the doctor pinpoint the precise location of the injury or problem.

Bone scans involve injecting a small amount of radioactive dye into a vein in your arm. The doctor allows the dye to circulate through your body for a couple of hours. Then, he will use a scanner, a camera-like instrument, to view the painful area. The scanner produces a picture either on a computer screen or on film. The radioactive dye will collect in the bones. The scan helps the doctor see any area of the spine that has an increase in blood flow and bone-forming cell activity. These changes could indicate a painful tumor, infection or vertebral fracture.

Discography also shows problems with the discs, a common source of serious chronic pain. In a discogram, the radiologist also injects a dye that shows up as opaque on an imaging scan into the disc or discs being examined. The doctor then performs a CT scan. The dye should illuminate any tears, scars or changes in the disc that may be causing pain.

In myelography, the doctor injects a special radiopaque dye into the spinal canal. This dye looks opaque on a standard X-ray, while the bones and tissues around it appear translucent. The dye can highlight a painful condition such as a herniated disc or nerve root compression.

Unlike other imaging tests, these three tests are invasive. Like a surgery, this term means that the doctor must enter the body to perform the tests. Invasive tests have some potential for complications, such as infection. Your doctor should discuss the potential for these risks with you beforehand.

Microfocal radiography and thermography. Some newer imaging tests allow doctors to detect damage such as deteriorated cartilage, joint erosions, inflamed soft tissues or synovitis (inflamed joint lining) at early stages, before these problems would show up on X-rays.

Microfocal radiography uses enhanced resolution scanning and a finer grain of film to produce a sharper image of the painful area. However, microfocal radiography equipment may not be found outside specialized pain centers. Thermography uses infrared technology to detect the heat that can be associated with painful inflammation. The scan can detect heat loss from the skin surface in a painful area, indicating inflammation. Neuropathic pain sometimes can cause a "cold spot" to appear on the scan.

Ultrasonography. A much less invasive scanning technique is ultrasonography or ultrasound, which uses high-frequency sound waves to produce pictures (called *sonograms*) of joints, muscles, organs and other parts of the body. The echo of the sound waves off the tissues produces the visual picture. These waves are harmless to the body. Ultrasonography commonly is used to view a fetus during pregnancy.

Doctors can use ultrasonography to diagnose a number of problems that may be causing pain, including ligament tears, subtle joint damage and more. Ultrasonography allows doctors to see inside the body without any invasive techniques, such as needles, dyes or exposure to radiation.

## Tests Involving Minor Surgery

The following tests involve having a small operation. Don't be alarmed: These tests only involve small cuts and usually can be done in a short time that won't require you checking into the hospital. In some cases, your doctor may do them in his office. Your recovery will be quick and any additional pain from the test should be very minor.

Arthroscopy. On the sports page where you read about your favorite pitcher having an

MRI scan to diagnose his elbow injury, you may also have read about him having arthroscopy or arthroscopic surgery. This is a very common, minimally invasive procedure – more than 1.5 million such operations are performed each year – that helps doctors diagnose or correct problems that cause serious pain in joints like knees, hips, elbows and shoulders. A slang term for arthroscopy is "getting scoped."

Your doctor may refer you to a surgeon (a doctor who specializes in performing operations) for arthroscopy or other types of surgery. The surgeon will make a small incision and insert a thin tube with a light at the end, called an *arthroscope*, directly into your painful joint. You may be awake during this procedure, but the area will be numbed so you won't feel anything. People undergoing arthroscopy usually don't have to stay in the hospital; they just have the procedure as an outpatient, staying for a few hours. Recovery from the surgery only takes a day or so.

The arthroscope is like a little camera, and it sends an image to a TV screen in the operating room. Your doctor sees what's going on inside your joint on the screen, and is able to move the tiny arthroscope around as needed. He may also insert other instruments to cut away ragged cartilage or to mend torn tissue.

A recent study questioned whether or not arthroscopy was needed in treating arthritis of the knee, because many doctors do the procedure for that purpose. Arthroscopy is simply a useful method for performing certain surgeries and in diagnosis. Some painful joint or

bone problems may not be easily viewed through imaging techniques.

Biopsy. While most people hear the word biopsy and think of cancer, a biopsy is just when a doctor removes a small piece of tissue to examine for clues to many other types of diagnoses. Biopsies involve surgery, but it's usually quick and the incisions (or cuts made during surgery) are often small.

Your doctor may need to perform a biopsy to diagnose diseases affecting joints, muscles, skin or blood vessels. In addition, doctors do use biopsies to remove growths to see if they are cancerous. A cyst or tumor (even if it is benign) may be the cause of severe pain in many parts of the body.

## What If a Diagnosis Isn't Clear?

There are so many problems that may cause your pain. Your doctor has a great deal of knowledge and resources at hand to help him figure out what is wrong with you, but he is only human. It may take some time before you and your doctor determine what is causing your pain.

Some of the reasons why your doctor may need some time to nail down your diagnosis include:

- Different diseases have similar or even identical symptoms. Your doctor may need to perform a number of different tests to figure out which disease you have.
- One person's disease may not be the same as another's. You may have a herniated disc in

your spine that is causing you occasional pain that sends you reaching for the menthol cream. Your neighbor may also have a herniated disc, but experience so much pain that she needs to go to bed for three days every time it flares. You have the same problem, but may not experience the same level of pain or the same exact symptoms.

- Diseases and injuries don't keep to a schedule. You may have osteoarthritis that has developed much faster than is typical, causing unexpected joint damage and a lot of pain. Your doctor may not be used to seeing patients with osteoarthritis who have your level of pain or movement problems. So your doctor may need to review all the symptoms carefully to determine your exact problem and its extent.

Your pain may continue while you undergo tests and search for the cause. Speak openly with your doctor about your concerns. Ask him if there is something you can take to ease your pain while he performs tests and rules out the wrong causes.

There are many mild, pain-relieving drugs that can ease your discomfort with few, if any, side effects. The most common is acetaminophen. Ask your doctor if it's OK for you to take acetaminophen now for your pain and if he has any guidelines for you for taking this drug. It's available over the counter and also in generic forms. Use caution, however; heavy acetaminophen use may be dangerous and lead to liver disease. Talk to your doctor about your options until a diagnosis can be determined and a course of treatment started. We'll learn more about this and other useful drugs for treating your pain in the next chapter.

## Developing Your Pain-Management Plan

Once your doctor has performed necessary tests and discussed your pain and other symptoms, hopefully you will have a diagnosis. Once you have a diagnosis, you have a name for the cause of your pain, and that's very important. You may have lived with serious pain for a long time without knowing why. You couldn't tell others, including your spouse, children, employer and friends, why you hurt. So other people may not understand the intensity and nature of your pain. They may think you're exaggerating or complaining unnecessarily, which can be frustrating.

That's why getting the right diagnosis is so important. You don't want just to treat the pain – you want to manage your pain while treating its cause. But once you have a diagnosis, you move on to Step Three, creating your pain-management plan.

What is a pain-management plan? It's not just a course of drugs; it's a comprehensive strategy for controlling your chronic pain on a day-to-day basis. Managing pain will require a long-term commitment from you. You will need to take your medications as prescribed. You will need to keep your body as healthy and fit as possible. You will need to get enough rest and keep your stress in check.

It's possible that your pain will never completely go away. But you can find treatments and strategies – not just drugs – that may make your condition manageable for you. You will find that some treatments and techniques work to control your pain and some do not. The strategies that work will go into your pain-management plan. Discard those techniques that don't work, but do so only in conjunction with your doctor.

Your pain-management plan can be something you keep in your head, or you can write it down and keep a document of everything you do. We suggest that you do keep a written record of your pain-management plan. Keeping track of the drugs or supplements you take, the alternative therapies (like acupuncture, TENS or chiropractic) you use, and the exercises you do will help you and your doctor get a clearer picture of what is working for you. Think of this document as a journal of your pain and your efforts to control that pain. Keep track of what you do and when you do it. Note the effects: Does the prescription drug your doctor gave you work to relieve your pain? Do you feel pain after your exercise routine? What kind of pain? How long does it last? Every detail will help you note patterns in your pain and identify techniques that work.

Your pain-management plan should have several components. It can include drug therapy, including prescription drugs from your doctor or over-the-counter drugs purchased at your local store. (We'll explain some of the differences between these types of drugs in the next chapter.) Your plan should include suggestions from your doctor about when you

should you take what drug and how much you should take.

Your plan should include more than just medications. Although you might like to take a pill for your pain and forget about it, most doctors would not recommend that approach. Many analgesic drugs have side effects, and they may not control your pain adequately by themselves.

To be successful, a pain management plan should be comprehensive. Pain may be caused by a physical problem, but your overall health and lifestyle habits can greatly affect your level of pain. Pain can get worse if you smoke, don't exercise or are overweight. Changing these habits can help you control your pain.

*Physical therapy* and *occupational therapy* are important options to explore as you and your doctor devise your pain management plan. These courses of therapy include consultation with a specially trained therapist. A physical therapist can create a customized exercise plan to improve your physical health or help reduce pain. An occupational therapist can work with you to adjust the way you do your everyday activities to reduce risk of injury and lessen pain. Either type of therapist may be able to fit you with customized *splints* or *braces* to place around wrists, knees, back or ankles to offer support, stability and help you manage pain.

There are many so-called natural or alternative therapies that you might try. These include herbal supplements, natural ingredients designed to help control pain, reduce inflammation or help you relax. (These remedies, while considered "natural," still carry risks. Chapter Seven will discuss this subject in depth.) Other alternative therapies for pain include acupuncture, an ancient Chinese pain-control method involving the insertion of tiny needles into your skin, or *chiropractic,* a more contemporary method of adjusting the spine to relieve pain and pressure.

Exercise can help build up your muscles so they can support weakened or damaged joints, and exercise can increase your flexibility so tendons, ligaments and muscles can function more effectively, with less risk of painful injury. Your doctor, in addition to a physical therapist, can offer you specific exercises to perform to ease your pain.

Pain is often worsened, or sometimes even caused by, stress and tension. Therefore, methods to reduce your tension can help control your pain. All of these important components of your pain-management plan – exercise, diet, healthy habits, relaxation therapies – don't involve drugs or chemicals of any kind. So these therapies can be a natural boost to your pain-control efforts.

While your pain-management plan should be comprehensive, drugs are an important component of controlling chronic pain. The next chapters explore the many drugs available to treat chronic pain and its sources. We will also discuss issues associated with drug treatment. These issues include how to use your medicine properly, cost of drugs, and how to differentiate between the various available treatments to find the best one for you.

# SAMPLE PAIN QUESTIONNAIRE

(Reprinted with permission of The Cleveland Clinic Foundation, Department of Pain Management)

**The following questionnaire is an example of the type of extensive, comprehensive pain survey your doctor might give you as you begin the diagnosis and treatment process.**

Outcomes Questionnaire: 1 3 6 month

**Patient Name:** _____ **Date:** _____

### 1. Where is your pain located? Fill in all that apply:

❑ Head          ❑ Hand          ❑ Pelvis

❑ Face          ❑ Chest          ❑ Buttock

❑ Neck          ❑ Upper Back          ❑ Genitalia

❑ Shoulder          ❑ Abdomen          ❑ Leg

❑ Arm          ❑ Lower Back          ❑ Foot

### 2. In general, would you say your health is:

❑ Excellent

❑ Very good

❑ Good

❑ Fair

❑ Poor

### 3. Compared to one year ago, how would you rate your health in general now?

❑ Much better now than one year ago

❑ Somewhat better now than one year ago

❑ About the same now as one year ago

❑ Somewhat worse now than one year ago

❑ Much worse now than one year ago

**The following items are about activities you might do in a typical day. Does your health now limit you in these activities? If so, how much?**

**4. Vigorous activities, such as running, lifting heavy objects, participating in strenuous sports:**

❑ Yes, limited a lot
❑ Yes, limited a little
❑ No, not limited at all

**5. Moderate activities, such as moving a table, pushing a vacuum cleaner, bowling or playing golf:**

❑ Yes, limited a lot
❑ Yes, limited a little
❑ No, not limited at all

**6. Lifting or carrying groceries:**

❑ Yes, limited a lot
❑ Yes, limited a little
❑ No, not limited at all

**7. Climbing several flights of stairs:**

❑ Yes, limited a lot
❑ Yes, limited a little
❑ No, not limited at all

**8. Climbing one flight of stairs:**

❑ Yes, limited a lot
❑ Yes, limited a little
❑ No, not limited at all

**9. Bending, kneeling or stooping:**

❑ Yes, limited a lot
❑ Yes, limited a little
❑ No, not limited at all

**10. Walking more than a mile:**

❑ Yes, limited a lot
❑ Yes, limited a little
❑ No, not limited at all

**11. Walking several blocks:**

❑ Yes, limited a lot
❑ Yes, limited a little
❑ No, not limited at all

**12. Walking one block:**

❑ Yes, limited a lot
❑ Yes, limited a little
❑ No, not limited at all

**13. Bathing or dressing myself:**

❑ Yes, limited a lot
❑ Yes, limited a little
❑ No, not limited at all

**During the <u>past four weeks</u>, have you had any of the following problems with your work or other regular daily activities as a result of your physical health?**

**14. Cut down on the amount of time you spend on work or other activities:**

❑ Yes
❑ No

**15. Accomplished less than you would like:**

❑ Yes
❑ No

**16. Were limited in the kind of work or other activities:**

❑ Yes
❑ No

17. Had difficulty performing the work or other activities (i.e. it took the extra effort):

❑ Yes
❑ No

During the past four weeks, have you had any of the following problems with your work or other regular daily activities as a result of any emotional problems (such as feeling depressed or anxious)?

18. Cut down on the amount of time you spend on work or other activities:

❑ Yes
❑ No

19. Accomplished less than you would like:

❑ Yes
❑ No

20. Didn't do work or other activities as carefully as usual:

❑ Yes
❑ No

21. During the past four weeks, to what extent have your physical health or emotional problems interfered with your normal social activities with family, friends, neighbors or groups?

❑ Not at all
❑ Slightly
❑ Moderately
❑ Quite a bit
❑ Extremely

22. How much bodily pain have you had in the past four weeks?

❑ None
❑ Very mild
❑ Mild
❑ Moderate
❑ Severe
❑ Very severe

23. During the past four weeks, how much did pain interfere with your normal work (including both work outside the home and housework)?

❑ Not at all
❑ Slightly
❑ Moderately
❑ Quite a bit
❑ Extremely

These questions are about how you feel and how things have been with you during the past four weeks. For each question, please give the one answer that comes closest to the way you have been feeling. How much of the time during the past four weeks:

24. Did you feel full of pep?

❑ All of the time
❑ Most of the time
❑ A good bit of the time
❑ Some of the time
❑ A little bit of the time
❑ None of the time

### 25. Have you been a very nervous person?

- ❏ All of the time
- ❏ Most of the time
- ❏ A good bit of the time
- ❏ Some of the time
- ❏ A little bit of the time
- ❏ None of the time

### 26. Have you felt so down in the dumps that nothing could cheer you up?

- ❏ All of the time
- ❏ Most of the time
- ❏ A good bit of the time
- ❏ Some of the time
- ❏ A little bit of the time
- ❏ None of the time

### 27. Have you felt calm and peaceful?

- ❏ All of the time
- ❏ Most of the time
- ❏ A good bit of the time
- ❏ Some of the time
- ❏ A little bit of the time
- ❏ None of the time

### 28. Did you have a lot of energy?

- ❏ All of the time
- ❏ Most of the time
- ❏ A good bit of the time
- ❏ Some of the time
- ❏ A little bit of the time
- ❏ None of the time

### 29. Have you felt downhearted and blue?

- ❏ All of the time
- ❏ Most of the time
- ❏ A good bit of the time
- ❏ Some of the time
- ❏ A little bit of the time
- ❏ None of the time

### 30. Did you feel worn out?

- ❏ All of the time
- ❏ Most of the time
- ❏ A good bit of the time
- ❏ Some of the time
- ❏ A little bit of the time
- ❏ None of the time

### 31. Have you been a happy person?

- ❏ All of the time
- ❏ Most of the time
- ❏ A good bit of the time
- ❏ Some of the time
- ❏ A little bit of the time
- ❏ None of the time

### 32. Did you feel tired?

- ❏ All of the time
- ❏ Most of the time
- ❏ A good bit of the time
- ❏ Some of the time
- ❏ A little bit of the time
- ❏ None of the time

**33. During the <u>past four weeks</u>, how much of the time has your <u>physical health or emotional problems</u> interfered with your social activities (like visiting with friends, relatives, etc.)?**

- ❑ All of the time
- ❑ Most of the time
- ❑ A good bit of the time
- ❑ Some of the time
- ❑ A little bit of the time
- ❑ None of the time

**How <u>true or false</u> is each of the following statements for you?**

**34. I seem to get sick a little easier than other people.**

- ❑ Definitely true
- ❑ Mostly true
- ❑ Don't know
- ❑ Mostly false
- ❑ Definitely false

**35. I am as healthy as anybody I know.**

- ❑ Definitely true
- ❑ Mostly true
- ❑ Don't know
- ❑ Mostly false
- ❑ Definitely false

**36. I expect my health to get worse.**

- ❑ Definitely true
- ❑ Mostly true
- ❑ Don't know
- ❑ Mostly false
- ❑ Definitely false

**37. My health is excellent.**

- ❑ Definitely true
- ❑ Mostly true
- ❑ Don't know
- ❑ Mostly false
- ❑ Definitely false

**38. What is your current work status?**
Fill in all that apply.

- ❑ Working full time
- ❑ Working part time
- ❑ Volunteer working
- ❑ Retired
- ❑ Vocational rehabilitation
- ❑ School
- ❑ Not working

**39. Since your last clinic visit, have you required any of the following?**
Fill in all that apply.

- ❑ Medication adjustment
- ❑ Hospitalization
- ❑ Surgery
- ❑ Emergency room visit
- ❑ Unscheduled doctor visit
- ❑ Urgent care clinical visit

**40. Medication Assessment**
**What drugs are you using regularly (more than twice a week)?**
Check YES or NO for each category.

**Anticonvulsants?**          ❑ YES ❑ NO

Amount and type: _____

_____

Antiarrythmics?   ❑ YES  ❑ NO

Amount and type: _____

_____

Opiates?   ❑ YES  ❑ NO

Amount and type: _____

_____

Benzodiazepines/
tranquilizers?   ❑ YES  ❑ NO

Amount and type: _____

_____

Antidepressants?   ❑ YES  ❑ NO

Amount and type: _____

_____

Non-steroidal anti-
inflammatory drugs?   ❑ YES  ❑ NO

Amount and type: _____

_____

Sleeping pills?   ❑ YES  ❑ NO

Amount and type: _____

_____

## 41. Alcohol Assessment

Within the last month, have
you used alcohol?   ❑ YES  ❑ NO

Type of alcohol. Check all that apply.
- ❑ Beer
- ❑ Wine
- ❑ Hard Liquor (i.e. whiskey)
- ❑ Not applicable

How many drinks a week do you consume?
- ❑ None
- ❑ Less than two drinks per week
- ❑ Three to five drinks per week
- ❑ Six to 12 drinks per week
- ❑ More than 12 drinks per week

## 42. Support System Assessment

Do you attend self-help meetings?
- ❑ Never
- ❑ Almost never
- ❑ At least once a month
- ❑ Several times a month

## 43. Treatment Helpfulness Questionnaire

How would you rate the quality of the following treatments received? One being of the least quality, 10 being of the highest quality. If not received, then leave blank.

Whole program
1   2   3   4   5   6   7   8   9   10

Medical assessment and treatment
1   2   3   4   5   6   7   8   9   10

Psychology assessment
1   2   3   4   5   6   7   8   9   10

Physical therapy assessment and treatment
1   2   3   4   5   6   7   8   9   10

Office visits with physicians
1   2   3   4   5   6   7   8   9   10

Medical diagnostic tests
(i.e. thermography, EMG)
1   2   3   4   5   6   7   8   9   10

**44. How satisfied are you with the infor-mation you have been given about your condition?**

- ❑ Very satisfied
- ❑ Satisfied
- ❑ Relatively satisfied
- ❑ Somewhat dissatisfied
- ❑ Very dissatisfied

**45. How satisfied are you with the treatment you have received for your condition?**

- ❑ Very satisfied
- ❑ Satisfied
- ❑ Relatively satisfied
- ❑ Somewhat dissatisfied
- ❑ Very dissatisfied

**46. How satisfied are you with the over-all medical care you have received at your pain management center?**

- ❑ Very satisfied
- ❑ Satisfied
- ❑ Relatively satisfied
- ❑ Somewhat satisfied
- ❑ Very dissatisfied

**47. When was the first time in your life that the pain problem for which you are seeking medical attention first occurred?**

- ❑ Less than one month ago
- ❑ Between one and six months ago
- ❑ Between six months and a year ago
- ❑ Between one and two years ago
- ❑ Between two and three years ago
- ❑ Between three and four years ago
- ❑ Between four and five years ago
- ❑ Between five and ten years ago

- ❑ Between ten and twenty years ago
- ❑ Between twenty and thirty years ago
- ❑ More than thirty years ago

**48. When did the current episode of the pain problem for which you are seeking medical attention first occur?**

- ❑ Less than one month ago
- ❑ Between one and six months ago
- ❑ Between six months and a year ago
- ❑ Between one and two years ago
- ❑ Between two and three years ago
- ❑ Between three and four years ago
- ❑ Between four and five years ago
- ❑ Between five and ten years ago
- ❑ Between ten and twenty years ago
- ❑ Between twenty and thirty years ago
- ❑ More than thirty years ago

**49. During the past four weeks, how many days have you missed work?**

- ❑ None
- ❑ 1-3 days
- ❑ 4-7 days (once a week)
- ❑ 8-11 days (twice a week)
- ❑ 12-15 days (three times a week)
- ❑ 16 days or more (daily or almost daily)

**50. During the past four weeks, how many days have you had to cut down on your time at work (arrive late or leave early)?**

- ❑ None
- ❑ 1-3 days
- ❑ 4-7 days (once a week)
- ❑ 8-11 days (twice a week)
- ❑ 12-15 days (three times a week)
- ❑ 16 days or more (daily or almost daily)

51. During the past four weeks, how many days have you been unable to meet work deadlines?

- ❑ None
- ❑ 1-3 days
- ❑ 4-7 days (once a week)
- ❑ 8-11 days (twice a week)
- ❑ 12-15 days (three times a week)
- ❑ 16 days or more (daily or almost daily)

52. During the past four weeks, which of the following terms describes your disability status?

- ❑ Not disabled
- ❑ Receiving disability payments
- ❑ Partially disabled
- ❑ Totally disabled
- ❑ Temporarily disabled
- ❑ Permanently disabled

53. During the past four weeks, which of the following terms describes your employment status?

- ❑ Unemployed
- ❑ Attending school/training
- ❑ Gainfully employed/full time
- ❑ Gainfully employed/part time
- ❑ Volunteer employment full time
- ❑ Volunteer employment part time

54. During the past four weeks, how many times have you received care in an emergency room or an urgent care center?

- ❑ None
- ❑ 1-3 times
- ❑ 4-7 times (once a week)
- ❑ 8-11 times (twice a week)

- ❑ 12-15 times (three times a week)
- ❑ 16-19 times (four times a week)
- ❑ 20 times or more (daily or almost daily)

55. During the past four weeks, how many times have you been admitted to the hospital?

- ❑ None
- ❑ 1-3 times
- ❑ 4-7 times (once a week)
- ❑ 8-11 times (twice a week)
- ❑ 12-15 times (three times a week)
- ❑ 16-19 times (four times a week)
- ❑ 20 times or more (daily or almost daily)

56. During the past four weeks, how many times have you undergone surgery?

- ❑ None
- ❑ 1-3 times
- ❑ 4-7 times (once a week)
- ❑ 8-11 times (twice a week)
- ❑ 12-15 times (three times a week)
- ❑ 16-19 times (four times a week)
- ❑ 20 times or more (daily or almost daily)

57. During the past four weeks, have many times have you been to see health-care providers (doctors, nurses, therapists, etc.)?

- ❑ None
- ❑ 1-3 times
- ❑ 4-7 times (once a week)
- ❑ 8-11 times (twice a week)
- ❑ 12-15 times (three times a week)
- ❑ 16-19 times (four times a week)
- ❑ 20 times or more (daily or almost daily)

58. During the <u>past four weeks</u>, how many times have you been prescribed medication?

- ❑ None
- ❑ 1-3 times
- ❑ 4-7 times (once a week)
- ❑ 8-11 times (twice a week)
- ❑ 12-15 times (three times a week)
- ❑ 16-19 times (four times a week)
- ❑ 20 times or more (daily or almost daily)

59. During the <u>past four weeks</u>, how many times have you had diagnostic tests (blood tests, X-rays, etc.)?

- ❑ None
- ❑ 1-3 times
- ❑ 4-7 times (once a week)
- ❑ 8-11 times (twice a week)
- ❑ 12-15 times (three times a week)
- ❑ 16-19 times (four times a week)
- ❑ 20 times or more (daily or almost daily)

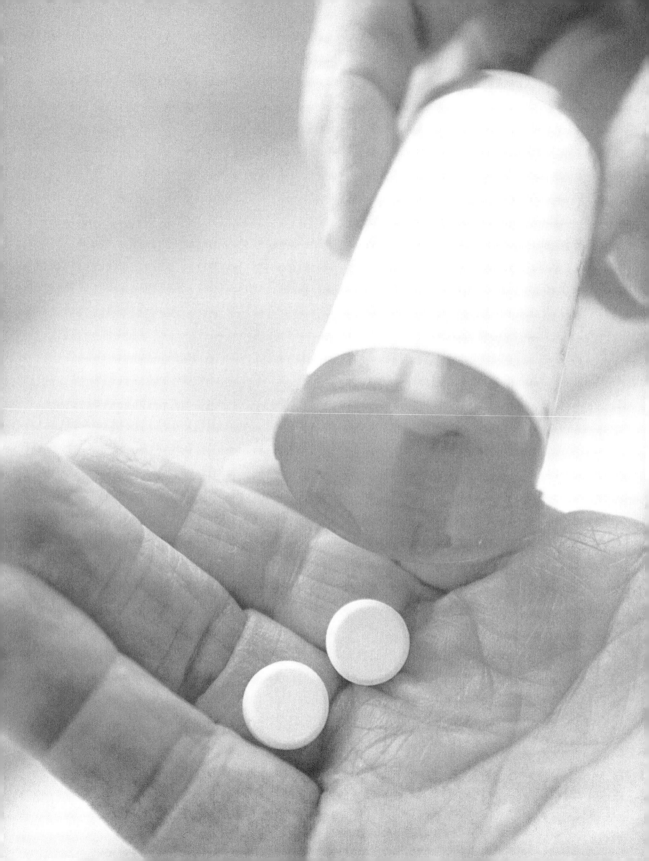

# Taking Drugs
# For Pain

---

3

# CHAPTER 3: TAKING DRUGS FOR PAIN

There are many ways you can treat your pain: drugs, "natural" treatments, lifestyle changes that can reduce or help you manage pain, new medical methods for curbing pain, and surgical treatments.

Treatment with a drug – or you may call drugs medicines or medications – is probably the most common approach to relieve chronic pain. Many drugs come in pill form, but your doctor may also give you shots or injections of pain-treating drugs. Some drugs are available over the counter, or without a prescription from your doctor. Others are available only with a prescription. Some drugs may be covered by your insurance, while others are not, so it's important to talk openly with your doctor about what he recommends and prescribes. Because some drugs used to treat diseases like arthritis can be very expensive, you'll want to find out about every option available to treat your pain. After all, why spend extra money if you don't have to?

In this chapter, we will discuss important terms about drugs, so you will know what you are taking and what you are buying. We'll learn what drugs are available to fight your pain and treat the underlying causes of pain. The good news is that there are thousands of drugs on the market today. Your doctor has the knowledge and experience to work with you to find the right drugs to treat your problem.

## WHAT IS A DRUG?

Drugs are chemicals or substances that affect the structure or functioning of your body. The drugs we are talking about in this chapter are *therapeutic drugs,* or drugs designed to treat problems or relieve pain. Doctors developed the first drugs from natural sources, such as trees, flowers or minerals. In recent history, scientists began developing more sophisticated drugs to target specific functions in the body in an effort to treat problems. Some drugs are *synthetic* or man-made versions of natural substances, even substances found within your own body, such as hormones.

Although there may be many drugs available to treat a problem or condition – for instance to reduce painful inflammation – you may find that one medication is more effective for you than others. Why? Even though some drugs do the same thing, they may treat the problem in a different way or have a different acting ingredient. To add to the confusion, some medicines are exactly the same except for their brand name. Your doctor can help you sort through the confusion to find the best medication to treat your pain.

As we discuss drugs, we will list the generic or scientific name of the drug first, and then list the brand names of the drug in italics and in parenthesis. Many drugs come in numerous brands; ask your doctor or pharmacist to help you decide which one is right for you. Generic or non-name-brand versions of many drugs are available. In most cases, there may be no difference except the price. In addition, some drugs may not be covered by your insurance policy, so check your policy carefully. If a drug your doctor prescribes is not covered, don't be afraid to ask your doctor and pharmacist if there are other options or generic equivalents that may be cheaper.

## Drugs: Important Things To Know

Simply put, a drug is any medicine you take to heal your pain or other problems. While you may hear the word "drug" used in discussions about marijuana, cocaine or other "street drugs," we're talking about helpful drugs that can treat your pain. Because pain medications can be serious and powerful, it's important for you and your doctor to work together to choose the right medicines for you.

Drugs can come in many forms: pills, shots, liquid drinks, creams or other formulations. As we learned in Chapter One, some drugs can help to narrow or even close the "pain gate" that allows pain signals into the brain. These drugs actually decrease the degree to which you feel pain. They "dull" the pain. Two, some drugs may work to heal the internal problems that are causing pain in the first place – such as inflammation, joint damage or infections. Three, some drugs are meant to replace lost fluids or to change malfunctions in your body that lead to pain.

In the last ten years, the number of drugs available to treat health problems has grown tremendously. There are thousands of drugs on the market and more on the way. Your doctor knows the right ones for you to choose from. As you and your doctor work together to find the right treatments for your pain, you may have some questions about how to take the drugs your doctor prescribes, what the drugs do and what effects they may have on your body. Be sure to speak up when you have questions about your drugs. It's important to take your drugs just as your doctor prescribes, and to know what side effects or cautions to be aware of. Ask your doctor to explain everything about your drugs during your appointment.

Drugs, whether ones that your doctor prescribes or ones that you buy without a prescription, should be only one part of that overall pain-management plan, albeit a very important part. A comprehensive pain-management plan includes not just drugs, but also regular exercise, a proper diet, stress control methods, and more.

Here are some important matters to consider as you and your doctor explore medicines to treat your pain or the conditions that cause your pain.

Prescription vs. over the counter drugs. An over-the-counter drug is a drug that does not require a prescription. Medical doctors, osteopaths, dentists and dental specialists, and psychiatrists can prescribe drugs. In some states, physician assistants and nurse practitioners, who often see patients in medical practices, can prescribe drugs. Nurses, chiropractors, psychologists and alternative healing practitioners cannot prescribe drugs. Over-the-counter medicines include common drugs like aspirin, ibuprofen or acetaminophen, medicines for stomach upset or creams for muscle pain. These drugs are available at your supermarket, drugstore or discount store. Many of these medicines can be very helpful for relieving mild, everyday pain.

When you receive a prescription drug, you will also receive specific written information about how to take the drug safely and effectively, and what side effects to watch for. You can ask your doctor, his staff or your pharmacist any questions you may have about the use of your drug. Over-the-counter medications also contain written information about the drug, its side effects and cautions about using it. But it's up to you to read this information and ask questions about how to use any drug safely.

If you find that you are taking over-the-counter medicines for pain on a daily basis, or often need to take the maximum, daily, recommended dosage for relief, talk to your doctor. If you are not finding adequate pain relief, he may wish to prescribe a medication that is stronger and more effective. In addition, there may be other lifestyle changes you should make to help control your pain.

Just because you can buy over-the-counter drugs at the corner store without a prescription does not mean these drugs are not powerful. If you take over-the-counter drugs for your pain, tell your doctor when you have your appointment. If you are taking prescription drugs, herbal supplements and over-the-counter drugs for the same pain, you may be taking too much of the same active ingredi-

ent. That's why it's important to tell your doctor about everything you take for pain.

Ask the pharmacist. This licensed professional fills the prescriptions from your doctor at drugstores or pharmacies. A pharmacist has years of specialized education and is the only person licensed to dispense prescription drugs. Pharmacies often have assistants who can answer certain questions about your drugs or your insurance coverage for these drugs. If you pick up your medicine at the pharmacy and have questions about how to take the drug or what side effects it may have, you should ask to speak to the pharmacist. Although pharmacists often seem busy and other customers may be waiting, it's important that you fully understand how to take your drug. Ask your pharmacist any question you have about your medicine. (See the section on p. 62.)

Active ingredients vs. inactive ingredients. The *active ingredient* in a drug is the chemical or substance that treats your problem. There may be more than one active ingredient in your medication. Some medicines are combinations of various drugs designed to treat more than one symptom, or one ingredient may ward off side effects (see p. 60) of the other ingredient.

In addition to the active ingredient or ingredients in the medicine, there are inactive ingredients, also known as fillers. These inactive ingredients should be clearly listed on the drug's packaging; if you don't see them, ask your pharmacist. These ingredients may make up the rest of the pill or liquid and make it edible or tasty, may provide a protective coating to keep the medicine from irritating your tongue or stomach, or may just act as a binder to keep the pill together.

Inactive ingredients shouldn't affect you. If you have allergies to certain foods or shouldn't eat certain foods, such as dairy, corn or sugar, you may wish to find out if the drugs you take contain these foods in their inactive ingredients. The drug might bother you or cause a reaction. This is rare, but it could occur.

Brand-name vs. generic drugs. Many companies can sell the same drug under different names, in bottles with different labels. Essentially it's the same thing. But the price can be very different. Think of a can of peas at the supermarket. Several companies sell cans of peas. There are even generic or "store-brand" peas. Are the peas different? Probably not. But the generic peas can be cheaper.

For some drugs, the generic form is much cheaper than the brand-name version. So you may wish to ask your doctor and pharmacist if the drug suggested for your pain comes in a "generic" form. Is it the same drug? The active ingredient – the chemical that does the intended job in your body – should be exactly the same. However, some other ingredients in the medicine, such as fillers or dyes, may be different. (See "active ingredient," p. 58.)

Some prescription drugs come in both brand-name and generic forms; others only in brand-name forms. Why? When companies develop a new drug, they have to invest their money in years of research and testing to create the drug. They recoup this money during the first years of sales of the drug, when they have an exclusive right to sell it. After a few years, this exclusivity runs out, and other companies are allowed to create their own versions of the same drug. If another company has not had to spend a lot of money to research and test the drug, it can create a form of the drug at lower cost and still make a profit. That's why generic drugs are cheaper.

Your doctor should know if the drug he prescribes for you comes in a generic form. If he does not mention this option, ask him or the pharmacist. Your pharmacy may ask you if you would like to have the generic form of your drug instead if one exists. Sometimes, depending on the drug and your insurance coverage, generic drugs may not save you much money. Look at your insurance policy to see if you will save money by using generic forms of drugs. The staff at your pharmacy should be able to find out quickly whether you would benefit from selecting the generic drug.

In addition to prescription drugs, there are also brand-name and generic versions of many over-the-counter drugs, like acetaminophen, aspirin and ibuprofen. You might see "drugstore brands" of these medicines at your local pharmacy. They can be much cheaper in price. But if you like a brand-name over-the-counter drug, you may not wish to switch to an unfamiliar product to save some money. It's up to you. Ask the pharmacist to help you compare brands if you're unsure. One way to compare these products is to review the active ingredients listed on the packaging. If the two products contain the same amount of the same medicine, they are essentially the same drug.

Refills of prescriptions. If you use your entire prescribed drug, whether it's a bottle of pills, a tube of ointment or a supply of liquid medicine, you will have to get a *refill* to get more. Your doctor decides how much medicine is included in your original prescription, including how many refills you may have. Some prescriptions have unlimited refills. You can get more medicine from the pharmacy whenever you run out. Others have limited refills (perhaps one or two). You will know exactly how many refills you can have when you first get the prescription. The prescription label or insert will state clearly how many refills are available. You may ask the pharmacy staff also.

If you run out of medicine and your prescription doesn't allow any more refills, you will have to make an appointment with your doctor or call your doctor to discuss it. Your doctor may not wish to prescribe any more of this medicine at this time.

Why? There are many reasons your doctor may wish you to use some medicines only for a short time. Once you have used a certain amount, if you don't find pain relief, your doctor may want to try something else. Drugs, as we learned earlier, can have side effects, so your doctor may not want you to take dose after dose of some drugs.

Some other medicines may carry the risk of *dependence* (see page 70). Dependence means that you have a need for the drug that is not healthy. You feel that you must take the drug or you cannot function. You may also build up a *tolerance* for certain drugs, requiring you to take higher and higher doses in order to obtain relief, and increasing the risk of unpleasant or dangerous side effects. Some medicines are very powerful and your doctor may worry that you will take too much, leading him to prescribe limited amounts at a time. Your doctor has good reasons to prescribe limited refills for particular drugs: your health and well-being.

If you use a drug, don't have any refills, but would like to continue using the drug, call your doctor. You should discuss the benefits and possible risks of continuing to use it. Your doctor may give you another prescription either for the same drug or another medicine. Or he may suggest other methods for you to relieve pain without using more of this drug.

Side effects and cautions. All drugs or medicines have side effects. This means you may have an unusual or unpleasant experience when you take the drug. These side effects can be anything from a rash to an upset stomach to unusual sleepiness or feeling "hyper." Even common, over-the-counter medicines may have side effects that are very noticeable.

Sometimes, side effects are minor. If you want pain relief, you may find the occasional side effect an acceptable trade-off. However, some side effects are very unpleasant or even dangerous to your health. These side effects may have to do with the particular drug or the necessary *dosage* required for adequate pain relief with this drug. Some people experience side effects that are as serious and painful as the problem the drug was meant to treat. In those cases, alternatives must be found. To avoid this danger, researchers constantly work to develop new drugs that treat pain with less risk of dangerous side effects.

When your doctor prescribes a drug, he should talk to you about possible side effects. Ask him what you might expect. Ask him what side effects should signal caution. In other words, if you experience certain side effects, you may wish to stop using the drug and contact him immediately. Cautions associated with drugs – these should be clearly marked on packaging of both over-the-counter and prescription medicines – are strong warnings not to take the drug in certain circumstances. You might also see specific warnings on the drug's packaging. These warnings clearly state what you should not do while taking this drug, such as driving or drinking alcohol. If you need help understanding these warnings or the written materials provided with any drug (these materials can be written in somewhat technical or medical language), ask your pharmacist.

Some drugs should not be used if you are taking certain other drugs, as the two medicines could cause a dangerous reaction when combined. People with certain health conditions might only use some drugs with caution, as their health condition might worsen by taking this drug even if the drug is for another, unrelated health problem. For example, if you have high blood pressure and get a cold, taking certain decongestants might be unhealthy. The drugs you are taking for your cold might interact with medicines you take to control your high blood pressure. Or, if you take other drugs, such as tranquilizers, it might be dangerous to take the decongestant for your cold in addition to the tranquilizer. These facts would be noted as cautions or precautions of taking the decongestant.

## Questions About Your Health

Your health is important. When you're in pain, you deserve attention for that pain and, if possible, fast, effective relief. To get relief, your doctor may suggest and prescribe drugs for you to take. Because drugs can be very powerful and even have side effects, it's very important that you take them as directed.

Drugs often need to be taken in a certain way in order to be effective and not cause problems in your body. For example, some drugs might cause stomach upset if you don't take them with food. Other drugs should be taken at certain intervals – such as every four to six hours – in order to work best. Some drugs should not be taken when you are also having any alcoholic drinks, because they can make you overly sleepy or woozy.

All of these facts are very important. You could hurt yourself if you take a drug improperly. At the very least, the drug may not work as well as it should if you don't take it as prescribed.

Your prescription will come with instructions about how to take the drug properly. Usually, there is a sheet handed out with the prescription with this information. The prescription bottle also may have instructions

## QUICK TERMS ABOUT DRUGS

**Caplet:** Another word for pill, except that caplets usually have a light, edible coating that makes them easier to swallow than normal pills.

**Capsule:** Small tube that holds tiny amounts of medicine. The casing of the tube is edible and dissolves in your stomach with water or liquid. The capsule allows you to swallow the exact right amount of medicine without tasting it (some medicines can taste pretty bad) or having it dissolve in your mouth.

**Implant:** A tiny device placed inside the body or under the skin that releases small amounts of medicine at regular intervals. Implants allow you to have medicine at regular intervals without having to take a pill.

**Injection:** A shot. A syringe or tube containing liquid medicine with a needle on the end that goes into your body. Your

doctor or a nurse usually gives you an injection of medicine for pain. This takes place in the doctor's office.

**Intravenous:** When medicine is inserted into the body through a needle into a vein. Doctors or nurses perform this procedure in a medical office.

**Ointment:** Another term for cream or topical agent. Can be gel-like or creamy. Ointments are rubbed on the skin.

**Pill:** Small, compressed ball of powdered medicine that can be swallowed with liquid or, in some cases, chewed and swallowed without liquid. Pills can be coated or uncoated. Coating may be used to keep pills from dissolving in your mouth, making them easier to swallow or keeping you from tasting the inside, which may taste bad. Coating may also serve to protect the lining of your stomach from the dissolving medicine.

---

printed on it. If you don't really understand the instructions (and they can be written in language that many people don't understand), you should ask for clarification.

Do not feel bad if you don't understand what your doctor or pharmacist tells you at first about medicines or any other methods you use to relieve pain. Your doctor may not

realize that you don't understand what to do unless you tell him. If you don't feel comfortable talking to your doctor about the drug, ask the nurses in your doctor's office or ask your pharmacist. Often, when you fill your prescription, the pharmacy staff will say, "Do you have any questions for the pharmacist?" Ask your questions then and

**Powder:** Some over-the-counter, pain-relieving medicines come in powder form. The powder is pre-measured and contained in small packets. You dissolve the powder in water and drink the medicine as a liquid. Powdered medicine may be harder to find in stores, but if you have trouble swallowing medicine in pill form, it may be useful.

**Spray:** Liquid medicine that comes out of a pump or aerosol (like a hairspray can) container. Spray medicines may be squirted up your nose, in your mouth or on your skin.

**Suppository:** A soft, dissolving capsule or pill meant to be inserted in the rectum. Usually, an applicator, or device to get the capsule into the rectum, is provided. Suppositories can release medicine into the bloodstream more quickly than drugs taken by mouth. They can, in some cases, also prevent or lessen stomach upset as a side effect.

**Suspension:** A liquid medicine that has the active ingredient suspended or contained in an edible liquid. You swallow a prescribed amount of the suspension using a measuring spoon, the bottle's cap or a small plastic cup provided with the bottle. Suspensions may be used for small children or for adults who have trouble swallowing pills for some reason. Not all medicines are readily available in liquid form, so speak to your doctor if you struggle to swallow pills and need a liquid medicine.

**Topical agent:** Also known as creams, ointments, salves or rubs. Smooth, paste-like medicine that you rub on. Topical agents contain all kinds of medicine, including antibiotics, analgesics and antihistamines. They should be used topically, or rubbed on the skin. They are not meant to be swallowed or inserted into the body unless the prescription says so clearly.

there! The pharmacist is busy, but not too busy to do his or her job and answer your questions. Your doctor, nurses and pharmacist want you to take your medicines the right way so you find relief and don't experience unnecessary side effects.

So don't be shy. Ask your doctor to explain what the medicine he prescribes does and how to take it properly. Ask your pharmacist to explain it again when you pick up the prescription. Tell your doctor about other drugs or treatments you use for various problems. When you talk openly with your doctor, he is more informed about your health, and you are more informed about how to improve your health.

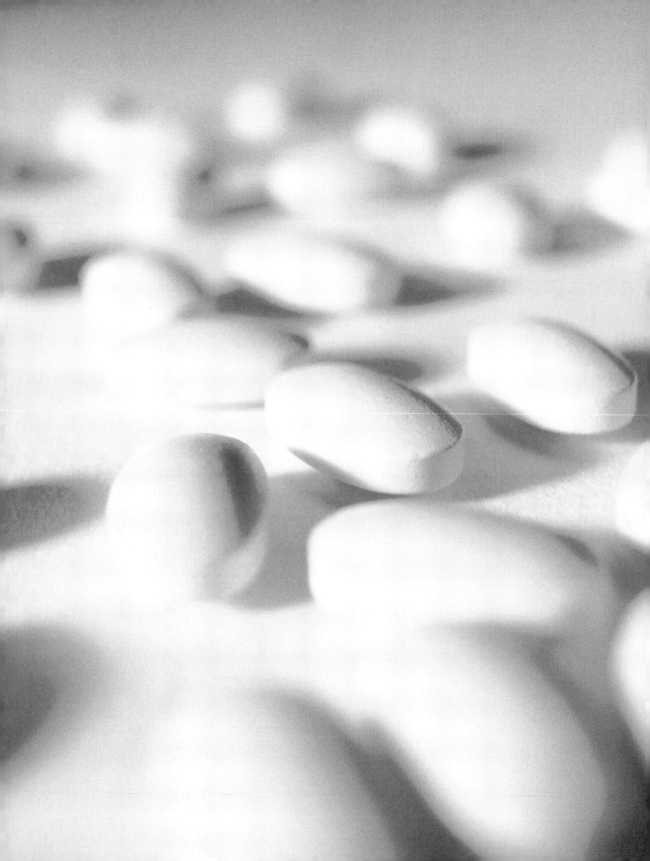

# Analgesics and NSAIDs

4

# CHAPTER 4: ANALGESICS AND NSAIDs

Now you know many of the different words associated with drugs. Having this vocabulary should help you better understand your conversations with your doctor and your pharmacist. It's very important that you know what drugs you are taking, and what different drugs do to help you.

In this chapter, you'll learn more about the many drugs your doctor might prescribe for pain. We'll also discuss some of the most common over-the-counter drugs you may be using for your pain. We will learn about how these drugs work to ease your pain or to treat the underlying cause of your pain. We will also begin to discuss side effects and other cautions associated with using these drugs.

It's important for you to be involved and aware as you begin using a drug. Your responsibility doesn't end when you swallow the pill or when the sting of the injection fades. You must take your drugs according to your doctor's instructions. You should stay aware of how effectively the drug works, and take note of any side effects you experience.

In this chapter, we will look at two of the most common classes of drugs used to relieve pain: analgesics and non-steroidal anti-inflammatory drugs, or NSAIDs. Chances are high that you have used one of these drugs or are using one now for pain relief. Some widely used analgesics and NSAIDs are available over the counter at a low cost, but other drugs in this class are stronger and require a prescription. In recent years, researchers have developed new drugs in these categories that relieve pain effectively but have less risk of adverse side effects. While they work in very different ways, medications in both categories can relieve most of the common causes of chronic pain.

## ANALGESICS

If you've ever used over-the-counter pain relievers, you may have noticed the term analgesic on the bottle. Analgesic simply means "pain-fighting." This is a group of drugs that reduce pain. They're used for many common ailments, from headaches to short-term illnesses like colds.

Analgesic drugs may not treat the underlying cause of pain, such as reducing inflammation or treating infections. They simply work to reduce your sensation of pain. Some analgesic drugs, such as acetaminophen, well known by brand names like *Tylenol*, also have *antipyretic* effects, or reducing fever or body temperature. Analgesic drugs are a very effective and important way to control chronic pain.

## Acetaminophen

When a medicine bottle says "aspirin-free pain reliever," acetaminophen is the drug you are probably taking. According to the American College of Rheumatology, the official organization of rheumatologists, or doctors specializing in the treatment of arthritis and other rheumatic diseases, acetaminophen is the first drug you should take for minor osteoarthritis pain. The daily dose should not exceed 4 grams of medicine. Higher doses of this drug could lead to liver disease.

Acetaminophen can reduce mild to moderate pain and reduce fever, but it does not treat swelling, redness or stiffness that may be associated with some chronic pain conditions. So your doctor might instruct you to take acetaminophen in addition to other medications to treat the other symptoms. If you take over-the-counter acetaminophen regularly for your pain, tell your doctor. It's not advisable to take acetaminophen for pain for more than 10 days without your doctor's supervision. It's important to tell your doctor the amount of acetaminophen you take on a daily basis.

Some brands of acetaminophen contain higher doses of the medicine in each pill. These brands' labels may read "extra-strength," but you should compare the amount of acetaminophen various brands contain. In addition, generic forms of the drug are sold widely in drugstores. Compare prices and the amount of acetaminophen contained in brand-name vs. generic medicines.

Acetaminophen is often combined with other, more powerful analgesics in one medicine. We'll learn more about these drugs later in this chapter.

**Common brand names:** *Tylenol, Excedrin Aspirin-Free, Panadol, Anacin Aspirin-Free* (*Excedrin Caplets* contain both acetaminophen and aspirin. There may be other over-the-counter brands that blend the two drugs.

Consult your pharmacist or doctor to know more about these medicines.)

**Cautions:** While acetaminophen, when taken in the right amounts, shouldn't have side effects, there are some things you should know. It's dangerous to take acetaminophen if you drink alcohol regularly. Regular alcohol consumption means about three or more alcoholic drinks (such as a 12 oz. bottle of beer, a 4 oz. glass of wine or a mixed drink containing 1 ounce of hard liquor) each day.

In fact, if you take more than one or two doses of acetaminophen at a time, it's recommended that you avoid alcohol because the combined usage can increase your risk of liver or kidney damage. If you find that you are taking large amounts of acetaminophen for your pain, you may be at increased risk of liver or kidney damage, so your doctor may wish to prescribe a different drug for your pain.

Advisors to the United States Food and Drug Administration (FDA), the official government agency that tests and approves all drugs (both over-the-counter and prescription) for sale in the U.S., urged the agency in September 2002 to require a stronger warning on packaging labels of acetaminophen products stressing that using this popular pain reliever improperly can lead to liver toxicity. So even though this is a very common drug (used by as many as 100 million people in the U.S. per year, according to the FDA), it's important that you take acetaminophen as recommended. If you have chronic pain and feel that you need to take acetaminophen often or in high doses, talk to your doctor about how much and how often you take this drug. He may wish to monitor your liver function or prescribe something else.

It's important to be honest with your doctor about how much beer, wine or liquor you drink on a daily or regular basis. Don't worry about him judging you. Your health is at stake. You might also think about curbing your drinking if you need to take medicine for pain often.

Some brands of pain relievers combine acetaminophen with other drugs, such as aspirin, antihistamines (allergy medicine), decongestants (medicines that dry up nasal congestion), diuretics (used to flush fluid build-up from the body) or others. Review the medicine you choose carefully to note all the active ingredients. If you only seek pain relief, you may not need a brand that contains other medicines. If you are allergic to aspirin, you may wish to take a brand that only contains acetaminophen. Aspirin and ibuprofen, which are explained fully later in this chapter, treat inflammation. If you only need pain relief, you may not need these drugs in addition to the acetaminophen.

## Narcotics

Some people need an analgesic more powerful than acetaminophen alone. Your doctor can prescribe pills that contain acetaminophen mixed with stronger drugs for more pain relief. The stronger drugs added usually are narcotics. Doctors often prescribe small amounts of narcotic drugs like combined acetaminophen with codeine or hydrocodone for severe, acute (short-term) pain, such as from a broken bone or a herniated disc.

Narcotics are derived from opium, which comes from poppy flowers. That's why these drugs may be called opiates or opioids. You may hear the term narcotics and think of junkies, dirty needles and illegal drug abuse. While some people illegally abuse narcotic drugs, these medicines have great value for people with serious pain. They are safe and effective when you use them according to your doctor's instructions.

For many years, doctors believed that prescribing narcotics for people with chronic pain was not a good idea. They felt people would have to take the drug for a long period of time to maintain pain relief. Doctors worried that these people would develop a dependence on the drug. (See "Narcotics: Can You Get Hooked?" on p. 70.)

In recent years, newspapers, magazines and TV news programs widely reported and discussed celebrities – including TV stars and football players who received prescriptions of the drug following injuries or accidents – who had become addicted to the commonly prescribed narcotic hydrocodone or others. These stories rekindled an old debate about the possible risks of prescribing these drugs for pain.

The newer, powerful narcotic oxycodone (*OxyContin, Roxicodone, OxyFAST, OxylR liquid*) caused an even greater storm of controversy after reports of robberies and illegal abuse of the drug (sometimes called "hillbilly heroin" by abusers and criminal drug traffickers). But hydrocodone, oxycodone and other narcotics have important, confirmed health value. Many people with severe chronic pain use these prescription drugs properly for effective relief. For these people, these drugs are necessary to live a normal life.

Today, doctors are more likely to prescribe narcotics to patients who have not found pain relief through other methods. Still, some doctors prefer not to prescribe long-term narcotics for diseases with chronic pain (such as arthritis or fibromyalgia). They may prescribe short-term doses of narcotics to treat a particularly bad flare of the disease, but turn to other drugs to treat the symptoms of these diseases.

How do narcotics work? As we learned in Chapter One, when a part of your body is damaged or inflamed, your nerve endings send pain signals to the brain, and the brain responds by making you feel pain and producing other defensive responses. Narcotic drugs interrupt those pain signals, so they never get to the brain. They cause this interruption by imitating endorphins, naturally produced chemicals that block pain signals.

**Common brands:** Acetaminophen mixed with codeine (*Tylenol with Codeine, Fioricet, Phenaphen with Codeine*), acetaminophen mixed with hydrocodone (*Dolacet, Hydrocet, Lorcet, Lortab, Vicodin*), propoxyphene hydrochloride (*Darvon, PP-Cap*), hydrocodone (*Vicodin*), oxycodone (*OxyContin, Roxicodone, OxyFAST, OxyIR liquid*), demerol and morphine.

**Cautions:** Possible side effects of narcotic drugs include constipation, weakness or unusual tiredness, lightheadedness or dizziness,

drowsiness, nausea or vomiting. These drugs also carry the risk of dependence with long-term use. Drugs containing narcotics should not be used with alcohol, as drowsiness, a common side effect of these drugs, could intensify. If you develop constipation while taking these drugs, your doctor might recommend an over-the-counter stool softener, fiber supplement or specific foods to increase regularity.

## Newer Analgesics

There is a newer opioid analgesic that may offer relief for people with moderate to severe chronic pain that is not relieved by acetaminophen alone: tramadol. Tramadol is available by prescription only at this time, both by itself (*Ultram*) and in combination with acetaminophen (*Ultracet*). Some pain patients find that the combined drug offers better relief than tramadol alone; however, this has not been medically proven.

Unlike many other opioid drugs, tramadol is not classified as a narcotic drug by most medical experts. Yet tramadol does carry a risk of dependence, so doctors will want to monitor your use of the drug carefully. Medical studies show few reported incidences of abuse of tramadol, but the risk still exists.

**Common brands:** Tramadol (*Ultram*), tramadol with acetaminophen (*Ultracet*).

**Cautions:** May cause side effects such as constipation, diarrhea, dizziness, drowsiness, increased sweating, loss of appetite or nausea. These drugs do carry a risk of psychological or physical dependence. With *Ultracet* or any other drug containing acetaminophen, there is

# Narcotics: Can You Get Hooked?

One of the important risks of taking narcotics for pain relief is dependence. Dependence on a drug is different from *addiction*. Dependence suggests that the person would experience withdrawal symptoms if they stopped using the drug, while addiction is a self-destructive, habitual use of the drug. Abuse of drugs is a serious problem that could be life-threatening.

People who have serious, chronic pain and do not have a previous history of substance abuse are at low risk of developing an addiction to narcotic drugs. However, they might develop a dependence on the drug, and they also might develop a tolerance for the drug, which means that they would require higher and higher doses for pain relief.

Physical dependence on narcotics is a real concern. According to the American Pain Society's 2002 report, *Guideline for the Management of Pain in Osteoarthritis, Rheumatoid Arthritis, and Juvenile Chronic Arthritis*, nearly all people taking opiates on a regular schedule for more than a week developed a dependence on the drug.

The risk of dependence frightens many people with chronic pain, leading them to avoid what could be a very helpful treatment. People can be weaned off the drug if necessary, taking a tapered or gradually lowering dose of the drug. So a tapered dose of narcotics might be used for a short time during a flare of pain, but not used for pain on a regular basis. Few scientific, controlled studies have been performed to test the effectiveness of narcotics on people with osteoarthritis or rheumatoid arthritis for pain management. But the studies that have been done on these drugs demonstrate clearly that they can be effective in treating this type of severe pain.

In addition, some people using narcotic drugs may experience reactions of disapproval from friends or family. Such disapproval might make a person uncomfortable about using the drug, or fearful that the drug is somehow dangerous or bad. Narcotic analgesics should be safe and effective when used according to your doctor's instructions, just like any other drug.

For some people with chronic pain, other drugs and treatments don't work. If pain has become severe and affects your quality of life or ability to do daily activities, you should discuss narcotics with your doctor.

Some doctors don't like to prescribe narcotics for chronic pain; others believe these drugs can provide necessary pain relief and promote better sleep for patients who badly need it. Even doctors who support prescribing narcotics for chronic pain agree that narcotics are only necessary for a small portion of patients, and should only be used as part of a wider pain- and disease-management plan. This plan should include other medication options, exercise, healthy diet, lifestyle changes and non-medical pain-relief methods (such as heat and cold therapy or water therapy).

When a doctor and his patient decide that a narcotic drug is appropriate, they do so only after the patient understands the risk of dependency and the expected side effects of these drugs. Some doctors require their patients to sign a contract that outlines appropriate use of narcotics. Here are some of the central issues in the debate:

## Why You Might Consider Narcotics:

- Narcotics are effective medications for managing serious, chronic pain.

- Many people with chronic pain don't need narcotics. But those that do should have the option for a trial period.

- The addiction rate from narcotics is approximately one percent. Addiction (compulsive, self-destructive use) is not the same as dependence (withdrawal symptoms if the drug is stopped abruptly).

- Less pain results in increased ability to perform basic daily tasks and could promote better sleep during flares.

## Why You Might Avoid Narcotics:

- When you use narcotics, you treat pain but don't treat the factors that cause it. Therefore, narcotics should be used only in the context of a thorough pain-management and disease-management program.

- Dependence is an expected result of treatment.

- Narcotics will dull pain, but not eliminate it. In other words, it isn't a "cure."

*continued on next page*

# Narcotics: Can You Get Hooked?

- Most people develop a tolerance to narcotics after a while – from months to years – so they must continue to increase the dosage to have the same level of relief. Along with a higher dosage comes an increased risk of side effects and dependence.

- Narcotics have unpleasant side effects such as mental fuzziness, constipation, nausea, drowsiness and itching.

- Narcotics may not work as well for some types of chronic pain as others. For example, although there have been studies demonstrating the beneficial analgesic effects of narcotics in severe osteoarthritis and many other conditions, there have been no studies performed in fibromyalgia.

If you do experience chronic pain that does not respond to other drugs or treatments, you should talk to your doctor about narcotics. Discuss the possible risks associated with using the drug. Weigh your feelings about your ability to live an active life with your current levels of pain and your feelings about using these drugs. If you and your doctor decide that narcotic pain relievers are an appropriate treatment, follow your doctor's instructions carefully, just as you would with any other drug.

a risk of liver damage. Tell your doctor if you drink three or more alcoholic beverages per day and take any drug with acetaminophen.

## Topical Analgesics

Topical analgesics are creams, ointments, gels, patches or sprays that you apply on the skin over areas where you have pain. These medicines are available over the counter. They may work for a short period of time in small, contained areas of the body, such as your lower back, knee, shoulder or hands. They do not provide long-term relief for pain.

Topical pain relievers come in three varieties: *Capsaicin, counterirritants* and *salicylates*.

Capsaicin comes from spicy, hot cayenne peppers. The capsaicin temporarily blocks the transmission of substance P (see p. 11), a chemical that helps send pain messages from the damaged body part to the brain.

Counterirritants contain various natural oils, like menthol, camphor, oil of wintergreen, eucalyptus oil or turpentine oil, which create a short-lived sensation of coolness or heat on the skin over the affected area. This sensation helps distract your attention from the actual pain.

Salicylates are topical analgesics containing salicylic acid, the same ingredient found in aspirin. They stimulate blood flow, which may temporarily reduce mild pain and inflammation.

**Common brand names:** Capsaicin creams: *Zostrix, Zostrix HP, Capzasin-P.* Counterirritant creams: *ArthriCare, Eucalyptamint, Icy Hot, Therapeutic Mineral Ice.* (Another cream, *Menthacin*, contains a combination of capsaicin and counterirritants.) Salicylate creams: *Aspercreme, BenGay, Mobisyl, Sportscreme.*

**Cautions:** Topical analgesics are available over the counter and seem no different than hand lotion. But they are medicines, and there are some cautions associated with their use. If you are allergic to aspirin, do not use creams containing salicylates, as these could cause an allergic reaction. If you use any topical analgesic, don't use them with heating pads, cold packs or any other type of heat or cold treatment, as your skin could burn.

## Transdermal Patches

While pills are the most common form of pain-relief medication, some people experience problems with medicine taken by mouth. They may encounter side effects, such as severe stomach upset or nausea, or they may have trouble taking the pills at regular intervals. Some people may forget to the take the pills at the appropriate time for effective pain relief, and others may have schedules that make it difficult to do so.

For these people or others looking for alternative methods of taking analgesic medication, one solution may be the *transdermal patch.*

## THE SMELL OF PAIN-RELIEF SUCCESS

Some topical analgesics have a very strong scent. This odor may seem unpleasant to you, coworkers, friends or family. In some cases, the relief may be worth the stink! If not, or if you are going to an important event, such as a job interview or a wedding, and don't wish to give off the strong smell, ask your pharmacist to recommend a rub with less or no odor. They can be just as effective.

In addition, some topical analgesics create a strong burning or cooling sensation. If your skin is sensitive, this effect may bother you. If you find the product unpleasant once you have bought it and tried using it, return it to the pharmacy. Or, before you buy a cream, ask your pharmacy if you can open the tube and examine it first.

Transdermal means through the skin, and these patches contain analgesic medicine, usually the narcotic medicine fentanyl (*Duragesic*) or morphine-sulfate, that seeps slowly into the body through your skin. The patch attaches to the skin with an adhesive, almost like a simple bandage. The material that the patch is made of allows the correct amount of medicine to seep into the skin, where it is absorbed by the bloodstream. The patch lasts for about three days. After three days, you remove the patch and replace it with a new one.

Doctors prescribe transdermal patches for people with moderate to severe chronic pain. Most people who use transdermal patches have not found relief through analgesic pills or have some problems taking pills. While the transdermal patch may seem like a pain-relief method you stick on and forget about, these devices contain serious medicine. This medication carries some of the same side effect risks as other narcotic analgesics, and you should use the same precautions (such as avoiding alcohol) you would while using other narcotics. In addition, external heat sources – such as tanning booths, heating pads or electric blankets – can increase the amount of medicine that is released, causing too much of the drug to enter the body at once. If you use a patch, talk to your doctor about these risks.

We will discuss more methods for taking analgesic medicine without using pills in Chapter Six.

## NSAIDs: FIGHTING INFLAMMATION

One of the major causes of chronic pain is inflammation, which is characterized by combinations of redness, pain, heat, swelling and sometimes, decreased mobility. Inflammation can occur almost anywhere in the body, including on the skin, in the joints, internal organs, soft tissues and more. Terms ending in the suffix *–itis* indicate inflammation. For example, discitis is an inflammation of a disc of the spine, iritis is an inflammation of the iris in the eye and synovitis is an inflammation of the synovium or lining of the joint capsule. Arthritis is an umbrella term to describe diseases that affect the joints. Although the *–itis* in arthritis implies that there is inflammation of the joints, some types of arthritis, such as osteoarthritis, have little or no inflammation, just joint damage that can be very painful.

When a part of the body experiences injury or disease, inflammation is part of the body's natural response to the problem, triggering the process of healing and repairing of the damage. Inflammation can be very painful, and in some cases, inflammation can continue uncontrolled. Damage to the body can continue rather than healing as it should. That's why in cases of chronic pain that involve inflammation, it's important to reduce this inflammation.

There are a number of drugs that fight inflammation. Some of the most common medicines used to treat this symptom are nonsteroidal anti-inflammatory drugs or NSAIDs. You may also see the term "anti-inflammatories" to describe these drugs. NSAIDs include very common drugs like aspirin, ibuprofen (*Advil, Motrin, Nuprin*), naproxen sodium (*Aleve*) or ketoprofen (*Orudis KT*). Like acetaminophen, you can buy these medicines over the counter without a doctor's prescription. These drugs usually come in generic versions available at your drugstore or supermarket. However, some other NSAIDs are available only with a prescription. Some common NSAIDs are available over the counter but also by prescription at higher doses. The higher-dose, prescription versions usually have different brand names than the over-the-counter version. Some brands of medicine combine both NSAIDs (such as aspirin or ibuprofen) and acetaminophen to provide both pain relief and an anti-inflammatory action.

There are many different NSAIDs designed to treat the causes of chronic pain. Some medicines are applied for a wide variety of problems, but others are used for specific diseases, like gout, osteoarthritis or discitis. We will discuss specific gout drugs later in Chapter 5.

We know that inflammation is the body's response to damage or disease, and that inflammation can be very painful. Untreated inflammation may cause damage to joints and other organs. How do NSAIDs stop inflammation? NSAIDs work on the internal processes of the body to temporarily stop the production of prostaglandins. Some NSAIDs are called salicylates, meaning that they contain salicylic acid, which comes from willow bark. Aspirin is the most common salicylate, and aspirin was originally made from willow bark. If you have allergic reactions to aspirin, you should not take other salicylates or even herbal supplements derived from willow bark.

Children may also be at risk for a dangerous disease called *Reye's syndrome* if they take aspirin when they have a fever. Children who are experiencing pain should only be given medicines designed for children their age, or given the recommended dosage of standard drugs for children their age or weight.

NSAIDs commonly are used to treat diseases that involve inflammation of muscles, tendons and other soft tissues in the body. These are the soft-tissue rheumatic syndromes, including bursitis (inflammation of the bursa), tendinitis (irritation or inflammation of tendons), carpal tunnel syndrome (where a nerve in the wrist is compressed) or tennis elbow (where the epicondyle, a part of the bone where the muscles attach, is in pain). NSAIDs may reduce swelling and pain during a flare of these diseases, but they usually are given only as part of a comprehensive pain-management plan.

One serious drawback of NSAIDs is that they may cause serious stomach upset or gastrointestinal problems, such as ulcers, particularly if a person uses NSAIDs in high doses or over a long period of time. Serious gastrointestinal bleeding may occur. This risk, and possible counteractions and precautions you can take, are explained in the next section.

**Common brands:** Diclofenac potassium (*Cataflam*), diclofenac sodium (*Voltaren, Voltaren XR*), diclofenac sodium with misoprostol (*Arthrotec*), diflusinal (*Dolobid*), etodolac (*Lodine, Lodine XL*), fenoprofen calcium (*Nalfon*), flurbiprofen (*Ansaid*), ibuprofen (*Advil, Motrin, Motrin IB, Nuprin*), indomethacin (*Indocin, Indocin SR*), ketoprofen (*Actron, Orudis, Orudis KT, Oruvail*), meclofenamate sodium (*Meclomen*), mefenamic acid (*Ponstel*), meloxicam (*Mobic*), nabumetone (*Relafen*), naproxen (*Naprosyn, Naprelan*), naproxen sodium (*Anaprox, Aleve*), oxaprozin

(*Daypro*), piroxicam (*Feldene*), sulindac (*Clinoril*), tolmetin sodium (*Tolectin*).

**Salicylates:** Aspirin (*Anacin, Ascriptin, Bayer, Bufferin, Ecotrin, Excedrin tablets*), choline and magnesium salicylates (*CMT, Tricosal, Trilisate*), choline salicylate (*Arthropan*), magnesium salicylate (*Arthritab, Bayer Select, Doan's Pills, Magan, Mobidin, Mobogesic*), salsalate (*Amigesic, Anaflex 750, Disalcid, Marthritic, Mono-Gesic, Salflex, Salsitab*), sodium salicylate.

**Cautions:** For all traditional NSAIDs, the side effects are similar. They include abdominal or stomach cramps, pain or discomfort; diarrhea; dizziness; drowsiness or lightheadedness; headache; heartburn or indigestion; nausea or vomiting. If you notice any severe side effects or if they persist, call your doctor.

## NSAIDs and Stomach Problems

Most NSAIDs stop the body from producing all kinds of prostaglandins in order to reduce inflammation. But not all prostaglandins induce inflammation; some serve good functions, such as protecting your stomach from irritation. So when you stop the body from releasing all prostaglandins, you also keep the good ones from doing their jobs. That's why many people who take NSAIDs over a long period of time or in large amounts for pain wind up with stomach problems. These problems, such as ulcers, can be serious or even deadly. So doctors and researchers sought ways to offer them pain relief without damaging their stomachs.

Some doctors may prescribe not only an NSAID (see the full listing of commonly pre-scribed NSAIDs in the previous section), but also a man-made prostaglandin replacement known as misoprostol (*Cytotec*). When the NSAID stops the prostaglandin that protects your stomach along with the one that causes inflammation, this replacement steps in to reduce the chances of irritation. Another drug, *Arthrotec,* combines an NSAID, diclofenac sodium, and misoprostol in a single pill. It's available by prescription only.

Another method of protecting your stomach is to combine an NSAID with drugs that lessen stomach acid. Your stomach produces acid through millions of tiny, specialized cells commonly known as acid pumps. The acid pumped out of the cells helps to digest your food, breaking it down in the stomach so it can pass through the digestive system.

Your body also produces an enzyme called COX-1 (COX is short for cyclooxygenase) that produces prostaglandins that help protect your stomach lining from this acid. If your body didn't produce these prostaglandins, the acid would digest your stomach along with the food. That's why NSAIDs, which block the action of COX-1, can lead to stomach damage, particularly in higher doses or when taken for a long period of time. Taking another drug that lessens stomach acid production can reduce your risk of stomach damage.

There are two kinds of drugs that work to lessen stomach acid production: histamine or H2 blockers and proton pump inhibitors. H2 blockers include cimetidine (*Tagamet*), ranitidine hydrochloride (*Zantac*), famotidine (*Pepcid*) and nizatidine (*Axid Pulvules*). Some of these drugs may sound very familiar to you; that's because after many years of being available only by prescription, many are now sold over the counter in lower doses and at a much lower cost.

Proton pump inhibitors are available only by prescription. These medications decrease the amount of acid produced by the millions of acid pumps in your stomach. Proton pump inhibitors often are prescribed for a disease called *acid reflux,* which involves stomach acid moving up into the esophagus, the tube that leads from your mouth to the stomach. This acid backup causes serious, painful heartburn and *erosions,* or tiny holes in the esophagus or stomach. Proton pump inhibitors (also known as acid pump inhibitors) include omeprazole (*Losec, Prilosec*), esomeprazole magnesium (*Nexium*) and lansaprazole (*Prevacid*). If taking NSAIDs has caused serious stomach pain or persistent heartburn, ask your doctor if one of these drugs may be helpful. Again, some are available over the counter while others are by prescription only, so cost may be a deciding factor.

## COX-2 Drugs

NSAIDs block the production of COX-1, and this action can lead to severe stomach problems. What if a drug was more selective, blocking only the production of the prostaglandin that causes inflammation and leaving the others alone? Researchers asked themselves the same question, and in 2000, developed a new class of NSAIDs called *COX-2 specific inhibitors* or COX-2 drugs. These drugs selectively stop pro-

duction of the COX-2 prostaglandin that causes inflammation. They have much less effect on the production of COX-1 so it can do its job, which may reduce your chance of developing ulcers and other serious stomach problems while getting the anti-inflammatory benefits of the drug.

In clinical trials, where drugs are tested on controlled groups of people with the specific health problem the drug is designed to treat, COX-2 drugs caused stomach upset, stomach pain and nausea less frequently than traditional NSAID drugs. Tests on the people who took the COX-2 drugs showed that damage to the *mucus,* or slimy, protective fluid, on the esophagus was less than with traditional NSAIDs. Normal doses of COX-2 drugs caused two to three times fewer symptoms of ulcers or ulcer-related complications, such as gastrointestinal bleeding or obstruction.

Although traditional NSAIDs, like aspirin, can provide protection against heart disease when taken in low doses, COX-2 drugs do not provide this protection. If you have had heart problems or are at risk for heart attacks (your doctor can go over the risk factors and your personal risk), your doctor may advise you to take a low-dose (81 mg) aspirin along with your COX-2 drug for pain.

In addition, cost can be an issue with these drugs, because COX-2 drugs are new to the market and available only by prescription at this point. They can be expensive. According to the National Institute for Health Care Management's 2002 report, *Prescription Drug Expenditures in 2001: Another Year of Escalat-*

## TAKE YOUR MEDICINE (BUT DO IT PROPERLY)

Remember, it's OK to ask a lot of questions about how to take your drugs. In fact, we recommend that you ask as many questions as necessary to understand what you are taking, what effect it will have on your body, and how you should take it. You don't want to take drugs incorrectly. If you do, they might not work, or you might have unpleasant side effects like an upset stomach.

If you use any drug that your doctor did not suggest or prescribe, even if you follow the label instructions exactly, tell your doctor that you are using these medicines. Just because you don't need a prescription to take a drug doesn't mean that the medicine isn't serious stuff. Any medicine can interact with other treatments you use (even for completely separate health problems other than your pain, such as high blood pressure, allergies or rashes) and cause side effects or damage.

You should also tell your doctor what herbal supplements you may be using. These include glucosamine, chondroitin, St. John's wort and many, many more discussed in Chapter Seven. These substances may be "herbal" or "natural," but they can contain powerful agents that may either interfere with or intensify the action of your drugs. Serious complications, such as bleeding, can occur from drug interactions. Using two treatments that do the same thing might put too much of an active ingredient into your system at once, causing problems. That's why you must tell your doctor everything you are using.

Keep a list of what medicines or other treatments you use, how much you use and how often, and take this list to your doctor's appointment. That way, you will be able to remember everything you have done and help your doctor create the most effective pain-management plan for you.

*ing Costs,* the average price per prescription of *Celebrex* in 2001 was $97.32, and the average price per prescription of *Vioxx* in 2001 was $85.44. Prices of these and other drugs can vary dramatically depending on changing supply and demand, manufacturers' costs, the particular drug retailer and other factors. As with any drug, check your insurance policy carefully to find out if you are covered, and talk to your doctor if the drug is not covered.

**Common brands:** Celecoxib (*Celebrex*), rofecoxib (*Vioxx*) and valdecoxib (*Bextra*).

**Cautions:** Same as other NSAIDs, except may reduce risk of stomach damage. COX-2 drugs may not offer the same protection against heart disease that traditional NSAIDs do, so if you take an NSAID (such as aspirin) for this purpose, COX-2 drugs may not be a good replacement.

NOTE: Recently, the FDA issued a warning for users of valdecoxib to stop taking the drug immediately if they develop a skin rash. This rash could be a symptom of a possibly fatal allergic reaction to the drug.

In the next chapter, we will look at more drugs used for treating chronic pain conditions. Some of these drugs attack the source of pain, rather than dulling your perception of pain. Many of these new drugs are the result of groundbreaking medical research conducted in recent years to identify the specific malfunctions in the body that leads to inflammation and pain. These drugs could open a door to a more active life for many people in debilitating chronic pain, a door these people once thought was closed forever.

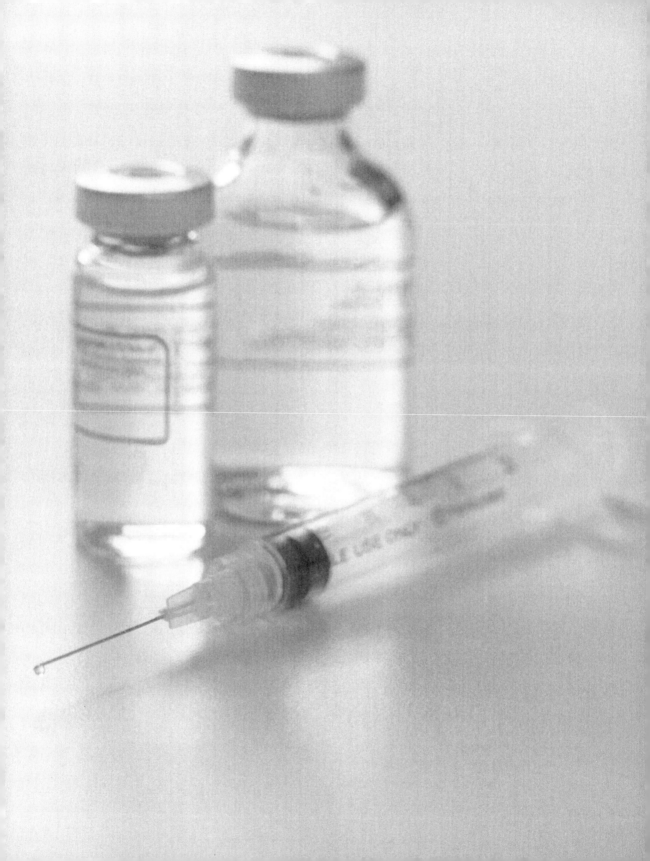

# Corticosteroids, DMARDs and More

5

# CHAPTER 5:
## CORTICOSTEROIDS, DMARDS AND MORE

As we have discussed, some drugs can treat the underlying cause of your pain, thereby reducing or even eliminating your pain. The diagnostic process discussed in Chapter Two will help your doctor pinpoint the cause or causes of your pain. With this information, he can map out a course of treatment, perhaps using some of the drugs discussed in the previous chapter or in this chapter.

In this chapter, we'll examine some of the drugs that fight disease by helping to correct the malfunctioning processes in the body that can lead to widespread inflammation and pain. We will look at some chronic pain syndromes that may need a combination of drugs to treat their many symptoms, and other types of drugs that may reduce pain for many people with chronic problems. We will also examine a therapy for knee pain that involves replacing the lubricating fluid often lost in osteoarthritis of the knee.

## CORTICOSTEROIDS

Other medicines you might use, available by prescription only, are powerful drugs that try to reduce the inflammation associated with some serious forms of arthritis and related diseases that cause intense pain. As we learned in Chapter Two, in diseases like rheumatoid arthritis, a person's immune system, or the system the body uses to defend itself against disease, goes awry. The body's immune system attacks itself, when it should be attacking viruses, bacteria or other organisms that make you sick.

In rheumatoid arthritis, known as an autoimmune disease for this reason, autoantibodies attack your own joints or, sometimes, organs like the eyes, lungs or skin. The result can be severe inflammation, pain and even damage to the joints or organs. To fight this inflammation – which can be disabling in some cases – doctors may prescribe strong drugs.

These drugs include corticosteroids, also known as *glucocorticoids* or *steroids*. Your body makes its own steroids, including cortisol, produced in the adrenal gland, located right above your kidney. The cortisol your body makes keeps normal internal functions running smoothly. Doctors developed a synthetic but much more powerful steroid similar to cortisol called prednisone to treat autoimmune diseases such as rheumatoid arthritis, Crohn's disease (a painful disease where the intestines and digestive tract deteriorate), lupus and many more. This drug helps to shut down the body's inflammation response when it does not "shut off" as it should.

The body needs to use inflammation in some instances, such as when you have an infection or have wounded yourself. This inflammation is a protective device because it jump-starts the immune system to heal the problem. The body releases chemicals to help fight the infection or other problem, chemicals that cause reactions like fever, swelling or pain. But unchecked inflammation can cause serious pain and even joint and organ damage. So doctors often prescribe corticosteroid drugs to reduce the inflammation and bring the disease under control.

Corticosteroids such as cortisone were considered a miraculous breakthrough when they were discovered and first used to treat rheumatoid arthritis in the late 1940s. The dramatic anti-inflammatory impact of the drugs seemed like the long-awaited "cure," even earning the scientists who developed the treatment a Nobel Prize for Medicine in 1950. But corticosteroids also may have serious side effects, particularly when used long-term or in high doses. (These side effects are described later in this section.)

Corticosteroids are not merely powerful drugs, but actually hormones that the body produces. When a person has a deficiency of these hormones, taking corticosteroid treatments may be less likely to cause side effects, but many people with painful, inflammatory conditions do not have a deficiency of the naturally produced hormones. So taking additional hormones through drugs like prednisone may lead to difficult side effects and long-term risks of diseases like osteoporosis (thinning of bones that can raise the risk of serious fractures) and avascular necrosis (death of bone). Corticosteroids slow down the formation of bone, so osteoporosis is a serious risk associated with long-term use of these medications.

Long-term use of corticosteroids, such as in rheumatoid arthritis or other forms of arthritis that involve inflammation, tells the body's adrenal glands (located near the kidneys) to stop making cortisol, one of the body's natural corticosteroids. (Cortisone, the first breakthrough corticosteroid drug, is a manmade version of cortisol.) If this person undergoes unusual trauma, such as an accident or surgery, the body can't produce the boost of cortisol that it needs to recover. So the person must have extra amounts of the drug. This can lead to greater risk of side effects and long-term negative effects.

Due to the side effects caused by corticosteroids, controversy surrounded the use of these drugs for many years. Until about 20 years ago, many in the medical community advised against using corticosteroids for rheumatoid arthritis treatment except in the most severe cases. That outlook has changed somewhat. Now doctors use these drugs effectively in controlled applications, often in lower doses than used previously for conditions like rheumatoid arthritis. Some people need a short-term, high (20-60 mg) dose of corticosteroids to treat particular conditions or a bad flare of inflammation. Other people respond better to long-term, regular use of a lower dose of the drugs.

A person who has taken high doses of corticosteroids for more than a few weeks cannot suddenly stop taking the drugs. If the person abruptly stops taking the drugs, he may experience confusion, withdrawal symptoms (such as fever, nausea or vomiting), disease flare or even collapse. So it's important to taper the dose gradually while the adrenal glands, which make corticosteroids in the body, build up their capacity to produce normal amounts of cortisol. This process generally takes about a month or two.

People often take corticosteroids in pill form. Some doctors may use a short-term series of pills called a *dose-pack* for a severe flare of symptoms. However, some people experience a sudden return of their symptoms as they take the pills in the dose-pack with lower amounts of corticosteroid. Many people take corticosteroids in smaller doses (such as 3 mg to 7.5 mg) over a longer period of time for controlling symptoms.

For some flares of a painful condition, such as back pain, arthritis affecting one particular joint, bursitis, tendinitis, tennis elbow or carpal tunnel syndrome, doctors may inject corticosteroid drugs into the body. Unlike some other drugs, you cannot give yourself these shots for flares of pain; you must go to your doctor for the treatment.

Doctors may give a person injectable corticosteroids through different methods, depending on their pain. One method is an *intramuscular injection,* or injecting corticosteroids into the muscle for absorption into the bloodstream. Two medicines often used for intramuscular injections are triamcinolone (*Kenalog)* and methylprednisolone (*Depo-Medrol).* Some people may be treated with intramuscular injections every two months rather than taking corticosteroids in pill form. This type of injection often provides excellent relief of pain and inflammation, usually lasting from one to eight weeks.

If a single joint is swollen out of proportion to other joints and is extremely painful, a doctor may choose to inject corticosteroids directly into the affected joint. Usually, the doctor removes as much fluid as possible (a process called *aspiration*) before the injection. Common joints injected with corticosteroids include knees, ankles, shoulders, elbows, wrists and knuckles.

Joint injections can be very effective at lessening inflammation and pain in a specific joint. This type of shot delivers a much higher concentration of corticosteroid directly into the joint. In addition, joint injections don't expose you to the potential side effects of taking oral corticosteroids. Unlike intramuscular injections, which may be given by any qualified doctor or nurse, joint injections require special training or experience.

Corticosteroid injections may relieve painful flares of tendinitis, bursitis or other soft-tissue rheumatic syndromes. These conditions involve inflammation of the soft tissue near a joint, rather than the components of the joint itself. Doctors can inject corticosteroids in the tissue around the wrist of people with painful carpal tunnel syndrome. Corticosteroid injections may also be applied at the base of a finger to relieve a "trigger finger," in which a finger does not open up normally, but suddenly with a trigger action. In some people who have fibromyalgia, corticosteroids may be injected into tender points, areas of great sensitivity and pain.

Some people may find relief through intravenous infusions of corticosteroids, or IV therapy. Doctors sometimes administer corticosteroids in very high doses through IV therapy, doses known as *pulses*. (The IV treatment may also be called pulse therapy.) These pulse doses may be up to 1,000 mg, sometimes given on three consecutive days.

IV or pulse therapy is effective at pain and inflammation relief, but results are temporary. Since the introduction of many other effective treatments in recent years (which we'll discuss later in this chapter), the use of corticosteroid pulse therapy has declined considerably. However, this treatment may still be effective in certain situations, such as acute flares of pain.

**Common Brands:** Cortisone (*Cortone Acetate*), dexamethasone (*Decadron, Hexadrol*), hydrocortisone (*Cortef, Hydrocortone*), methylprednisolone (*Medrol*), prednisolone (*Prelone*), prednisolone sodium phosphate liquid (*Pediapred*), prednisone (*Deltasone, Orasone, Prednicen-M, Sterapred*), triamcinolone (*Aristocort*).

**Cautions:** Corticosteroids can have serious side effects: weight gain, puffy face, high blood pressure, thinning of bones, less resistance to infections. Long-term use of these drugs can increase a person's risk of developing osteoporosis, the dangerous thinning and weakening of bones that can increase the risk of fractures. Long-term or high-dose corticosteroid use also can lead to cataracts, dangerous growths in the eyes that can damage vision; elevated blood sugar; insomnia; and mood swings.

Doctors often prescribe corticosteroids in small doses long-term in people with rheumatoid arthritis, limiting many of the side effects of the drugs while still being very effective at controlling inflammation. When people take corticosteroid pills, they may take a series of pills in a dose-pack with gradually lower and lower amounts of the medicine. This method of taking the drug is meant to wean you from the medicine, as your body might have a severe reaction to receiving a high amount of the drug then, suddenly, nothing.

## DISEASE-MODIFYING ANTIRHEUMATIC DRUGS

To fight the damaging inflammation present in rheumatoid arthritis, lupus and similar diseases, researchers developed powerful drugs that suppress various malfunctioning body processes or destroy abnormal cells that cause the painful problems in the joints. These drugs, as a whole, are called disease-modifying antirheumatic drugs, or DMARDs for short. This category includes newly developed, highly targeted and powerful disease-fighting drugs called *biologic response modifiers*. We will discuss these drugs in detail later in this chapter.

The most commonly used DMARD for treating arthritis-related diseases is *methotrexate*. This drug originally was developed in the 1940s for treating leukemia and breast cancer. In diseases like rheumatoid arthritis, methotrexate can kill abnormally behaving cells that lead to joint inflammation, damage and pain. Methotrexate is usually one of the first drugs given to people with moderate to severe rheumatoid arthritis, and has been a mainstay of treatment of this disease for many years.

Like cancer, in rheumatoid arthritis and similar inflammatory forms of arthritis, cells in joints do not behave normally. So the idea of killing abnormally dividing cells that may be leading to joint damage and pain makes sense. However, cancer and arthritis are two very different diseases. In cancer, if you kill 99 percent of the cancerous cells, the remaining one percent will continue to divide and cause disease, eventually returning the person to the same level of illness. But in rheumatoid arthritis, killing most of the abnormal cells can provide great pain relief for the person. So much lower amounts of methotrexate are needed to treat rheumatoid arthritis – often less than one tenth as much as is used to treat cancer. That's important, because methotrexate can have serious side effects, including liver damage, increasing susceptibility to infection, causing mouth sores and hair loss, and even causing a form of pneumonia.

Like corticosteroids, many people with painful, chronic, inflammatory diseases find relief from long-term, low doses of methotrexate (the typical dose is 7.5 mg to 15 mg per week in three doses, or 10 mg per week in a single dose), while only a small percentage of people need higher doses.

The development of DMARDs was another major breakthrough in the fight against arthritis-related diseases, which can cause serious chronic pain and disability. Like methotrexate, most DMARDs (pronounced DEE-mards) originally were used to treat other serious diseases before being used for rheumatoid arthritis, ankylosing spondylitis, psoriatic arthritis (a painful disease that includes skin rash and joint pain), Crohn's disease or others. But many of these drugs appear to help people who once felt beyond help, not only easing their pain but also stopping these *degenerative* (or worsening over time) diseases and the damage they cause to body parts.

Doctors may prescribe one DMARD or more than one in combination. They may prescribe one DMARD for a time then have you switch to another. Why? Every person's disease responds differently to these drugs, and it may take time to find the right drug or combination of drugs for your problem. Resistance to one DMARD could develop, and your doctor would have to prescribe another drug. In clinical tests, DMARDs have shown to delay the progression of disease, alter the natural course of the disease, prevent further damage and control chronic pain caused by the disease.

DMARDs are serious, powerful drugs that require frequent monitoring by your doctor, including blood or urine tests (see p. 35). Risks may include liver damage, high blood pressure, increased risk of infections and other potentially life-threatening side effects. Although DMARDs can treat the underlying malfunction that is causing the disease, if the disease includes inflammation as a symptom (as diseases like rheumatoid arthritis and ankylosing spondylitis do), you might take an NSAID or COX-2 drug along with your DMARD.

Ideally, a doctor should prescribe methotrexate or other DMARDs once he determines a diagnosis of rheumatoid arthritis or other disease requiring this type of drug, and before any joint erosions or damage appear on X-rays.

**Common brands:** Auronafin or oral gold (*Ridaura*), azathioprine (*Imuran*), cyclophosphamide (*Cytoxan*), cyclosporine (*Neoral, Sandimmune*), hydroxychloroquine sulfate (*Plaquenil*), leflunomide (*Arava*), methotrexate (*Rheumatrex, Trexall*), minocycline (*Minocin*), penicillamine (*Cuprimine, Depen*), sulfasalazine (*Azulfidine, Azulfidine EN-Tabs*), aurothioglucose (injectable *Solganal*), gold sodium thiomalate (*Myochrysine*). NOTE: Minocycline is technically an antibiotic, not a DMARD, although it is used along with DMARDs in treating rheumatoid arthritis and similar diseases.

**Cautions:** DMARDs may have serious side effects, including rashes, ulcers, diarrhea, kidney or liver problems, fever, dizziness, nausea or vomiting, pain and more. People using DMARDs may require frequent monitoring by their doctor.

## Biologic Response Modifiers

Biologic response modifiers (or BRMs) are an even newer class of disease-fighting drugs that can treat the malfunctioning body processes that lead to diseases like rheumatoid arthritis, lupus or Crohn's disease, the painful, chronic intestinal disorder. BRMs target specific chemicals that may be causing unchecked inflammation and suppress their production.

These drugs often provide astonishing levels of relief in some people who had almost lost hope that they would ever experience less pain and increased mobility. The four current BRMs on the market are etanercept (*Enbrel*), infliximab (*Remicade*), anakinra (*Kineret*) and adalimumab (*Humira*). More drugs in this category are in clinical trial stages now and may be approved for use in the future.

How do these drugs work? They inhibit or block the production of *cytokines*, substances in the body's immune system. Cytokines, in normal circumstances, fight disease. In people with diseases like rheumatoid arthritis, the immune system may continue to produce cytokines. This unchecked cytokine production may lead to inflammation that in turn leads to pain, joint damage and lost function or mobility. The biologic response modifiers etanercept, infliximab and adalimumab work in different ways to stop the production of a cytokine called *tumor necrosis factor,* or TNF, to stop inflammation and hopefully, prevent further damage. Another biologic response modifier, anakinra, blocks another inflammation-causing cytokine called *interleukin-1*. More drugs in this category are in the testing stages now.

These drugs cannot repair joint damage that has already occurred. But for many people, these drugs can reduce symptoms and restore some ability to perform daily functions. Many people who take these drugs experience dramatic relief of pain and improved mobility.

While these may seem like miracle drugs for many people, biologic response modifiers do affect the immune system. Therefore, people using these drugs potentially may be at greater risk of infections. You and your doctor should not begin your BRM therapy during an active infection, and may wish to modify your dose if you develop an infection of some kind. If you develop an infection while receiving this therapy, you should notify your doctor immediately to receive treatment for it.

Etanercept, anakinra and adalimumab are given by injection. Etanercept is injected twice weekly in 25 mg doses, underneath the skin in the thigh, abdomen or upper arm. You can either inject the drug yourself or ask someone else to do it for you. You must mix liquid into a vial containing the drug in powdered form. You must follow specific preparation and storage instructions for all of these drugs. Etanercept, for example, must be refrigerated because the natural protein in the drug can deteriorate at room temperature and become ineffective. Detailed information about how to prepare and store these medicines will be provided by your doctor and he will teach you how to administer the drug properly.

Anakinra is injected in a single, daily 100 mg dose underneath the skin in the thigh, abdomen or upper arm. Anakinra, like etanercept, must be refrigerated prior to use. Anakinra comes in pre-filled syringes and you can inject yourself. In addition, anakinra's manufacturer can provide a self-injection device called *SimpleJect*™ to help you. You should also talk to your doctor about how to administer the drug. Anakinra should not be used with TNF inhibitors.

Adalimumab, just approved in early 2003, is available in single-use, 1 ml, pre-filled glass syringes or 2 ml glass vials for subcutaneous (under the skin) self-injections. Adalimumab can be used in combination with methotrexate or other DMARDs.

Infliximab is given by an intravenous (IV) infusion, either at a hospital, an outpatient clinic, your doctor's office or in your home with the help of a home-care nurse. This is a two-hour procedure. Dose is based on your body weight, usually between 200 to 400 mg per dose. The first dose is repeated at 2 and 6 weeks, then given once every 8 weeks after that. Infliximab is only approved for use in combination with methotrexate at this time.

**Common brands:** Adalimumab (*Humira*), anakinra (*Kineret*), etanercept (*Enbrel*), infliximab (*Remicade*).

**Cautions:** When taking any of these drugs, your doctor will monitor your progress and reactions to the drug. You may experience irritation or redness around the place of the injection or IV needle insertion. Serious infections have been reported in some patients using TNF-blockers. People with active infections should not start treatment with these drugs, and those who develop an infection while using the treatments should be monitored closely by their doctor.

With etanercept, you may also experience pain or burning in the throat or a stuffy nose, as if you had a cold. With infliximab, you may experience abdominal pain, cough, dizziness, headache, muscle pain, nasal congestion or runny nose, nausea, shortness of breath, sore throat, tightness in the chest, unusual tiredness, vomiting or wheezing. With anakinra, you may experience reactions around the infusion site, such as redness, swelling, pain or bruising, as well as a runny or stuffy nose, sore throat, headache, low white blood cell or platelet count.

A small percentage of people taking anakinra developed serious infections, such as pneumonia. The percentage may have been higher in people who also had asthma.

## OTHER DRUGS FOR CHRONIC PAIN

Some chronic pain conditions may require specific drugs that address pain and the cause of the pain. In addition, some drugs developed to treat disorders not related to pain – such as seizures or irregular heartbeat – may have some pain-relief benefits as well.

### Gout Drugs

Gout, which we learned about in Chapter One, is a disease caused by a build-up of uric acid crystals in the body. There are a number of drugs that either can help reduce the uric acid build-up or help your body flush the uric acid more effectively.

Gout is terribly painful. People experiencing a gout flare may not be able to walk on the affected limb, keeping them from work and other daily activities. A joint affected by gout can be swollen, red and extremely sensitive to any touch (even a mild breeze). Gout attacks can happen suddenly, and should be treated immediately. If gout persists or reoccurs over a long time, a person might develop *tophi,* or solidified deposits of uric acid crystal. Tophi are firm, swollen nodules that can appear under the skin, often visible externally, in the fingers, toes or other areas.

Gout is one of the few chronic pain conditions that can truly be linked to diet, although this is not the only factor that plays a role in the development of gout. People with gout should avoid certain foods that are high in purines and should watch their consumption of alcohol. This dietary plan may help lower the amount of uric acid in the person's body and lessen the risk of a gout attack. In addition, proper consumption of water or other non-alcoholic, non-caffeinated beverages will help the person's kidneys flush the uric acid out of the body so it does not build up and form crystals. In the case of painful gout, prevention may be possible.

If you have a gout attack, it's important to treat the pain and inflammation quickly to find relief. You can also treat the underlying cause of the disease through one of several effective drugs. Some people produce too much uric acid, leading to the build-up that causes gout. For these people, a drug called allopurinol (*Lopurin, Zyloprim*) slows the body's production of uric acid. Other people with gout don't excrete uric acid efficiently, so it builds up in the body. For these people, the drugs sulfinpyrazone (*Anturane*) and probenecid (*Benemid, Probalan*) help increase the amount of uric acid flushed out by urination.

Because gout is an inflammation of the joint, an anti-inflammatory drug is often used as well. While your doctor may prescribe one of the NSAIDs listed on p. 75–76, another anti-inflammatory drug, colchicine, can relieve the symptoms of the gout flare, such as swelling and pain, and help prevent future attacks. A mixture of colchicine and probenecid in one pill is also available.

**Common brands:** Allopurinol (*Lopurin, Zyloprim*), colchicine, probenecid (*Benemid, Probalan*), probenecid and colchicine combined (*ColBenemid, Col-Probenecid, Proben-C*), sulfinpyrazone (*Anturane*).

**Cautions:** Drugs may have various side effects, including skin rash, itching, diarrhea, nausea or vomiting, stomach pain, headache and more. Some of these drugs may interfere with other drugs you take for unrelated health problems, so discuss your other medications with your doctor.

## Drugs for Fibromyalgia

Fibromyalgia, which we also learned about in Chapter One, includes various symptoms, such as widespread muscle pain and tenderness in various points throughout the body. Some people with fibromyalgia experience debilitating pain and sensitivity to the slightest touch or pressure. These symptoms can ruin the person's ability to live a normal life or work. People with fibromyalgia also often have extreme fatigue and sleep problems, creating a vicious cycle. They hurt, so they can't sleep; they can't sleep, so their body can't re-energize itself.

Why does this happen? It's hard to say. But we know that your body must have deep, restorative sleep – known as *REM sleep* or delta sleep – in order to restore itself and function well the next day. Some studies suggest that people with fibromyalgia sleep, but do not sleep deeply or long enough. Because they do not get the proper amount of REM sleep, their bodies do not restore themselves and they feel achy, fatigued and aggravated the next day.

Because the medical community has only recognized fibromyalgia for the past 20 years – and there are still medical professionals who do not recognize or understand the nature of the disease – little is known about why fibromyalgia occurs or how to effectively treat it with drugs. Studies conducted in the past few years and those going on right now may reveal much about the cause of the disease, leading to effective drug treatments.

Some drugs for the specific treatment of fibromyalgia are in the research and development phase, but at this time, the only drugs used to treat fibromyalgia are drugs currently approved and used for other health disorders. However, many effective drugs used to treat rheumatoid arthritis, for example, originally were used to treat other diseases such as cancer. So existing drugs can be useful for treating fibromyalgia, while research for new, fibromyalgia-specific drugs continues.

Researchers believe that one probable cause of fibromyalgia is that the person produces too much substance P (see p. 11), although the reason for this overproduction is unknown. Too much substance P might intensify the person's response to pain, causing them to perceive normal touches or pressures as terribly painful.

People with fibromyalgia might also have an abnormal production of serotonin, a chemical that regulates the way the brain controls pain and moods. Some research has shown that people with fibromyalgia either have low amounts of serotonin or process serotonin poorly. Not having enough serotonin may cause poor sleep, one of the most common symptoms of fibromyalgia.

Decreased serotonin production may also lead to a change in the way substance P is produced or released in people with fibromyalgia. For them, when a pain stimulus occurs, the decreased serotonin levels cause the pain messages traveling to the brain to become more intense or pronounced than the stimulus – such as a light touch – would merit. So someone with fibromyalgia would perceive something that might not cause pain in most people as very painful. A lack of serotonin may also lead to a change in the production of hormones in the brain known as HPA (hypothalamic-pituitary-adrenal) hormones, which regulate our response to stress, and the production of growth hormones, which also play a role in deep, restorative sleep.

Despite new research, at this time, there is no definitive evidence pointing to what causes fibromyalgia. Therefore, there are no drugs available to treat the root cause of the disease. In this case, doctors can only treat the symptoms with other drugs and hope that the person finds some relief. Other than pain and tenderness, most people with fibromyalgia experience sleep problems, fatigue and emotional depression. Therefore, doctors often prescribe drugs to treat those particular symptoms.

Antidepressants and anti-anxiety medicines, usually prescribed in lower-than-normal doses, can help the person with fibromyalgia sleep better and ease depression. Doctors may prescribe these drugs for chronic back pain as well. This group of medicines includes tricyclic antidepressants, selective serotonin reuptake inhibitors and benzodiazepines.

In addition, muscle relaxants might ease the muscle tension and pain common in fibromyalgia, and also promote sleep. Gentle sleep medications can also help the person with fibromyalgia get a restful night's sleep, allowing them to restore their energy and feel better the next day.

Many people with fibromyalgia take an effective analgesic for their pain. If you have fibromyalgia, you should ask your doctor if regular doses of an analgesic such as acetaminophen would be helpful and safe for you. Repeated doses of acetaminophen, as we learned earlier, carry risks. So talk to your doctor before using acetaminophen regularly for your pain.

Another treatment option for chronic fibromyalgia pain is low-dose narcotics, or perhaps the newer, non-narcotic opioid drug tramadol (see p. 69). These drugs might relieve pain for people who do not find adequate relief from antidepressants, muscle relaxants or sleep medications. People with fibromyalgia may wish to take the analgesics in addition to their other medications rather than in place of them.

As we discussed in the last chapter, some doctors do not support the use of narcotic analgesics for people with chronic pain conditions, including fibromyalgia, although these views may be changing. The best step is to talk openly with your doctor about your pain and what options exist to relieve it. Again, all drugs can have serious side effects if used improperly or unnecessarily, so trust his judgment.

Recent studies may suggest a connection between fibromyalgia and lowered production of the hormone cortisol, which we discussed earlier in this chapter. While this connection is not yet proven, people with lowered production of cortisol often experience similar symptoms to people with fibromyalgia. Some doctors feel that if this link proves to be true, use of corticosteroid drugs may be helpful for people with fibromyalgia. However, at this time, people with fibromyalgia usually do not take corticosteroids except in the form of tender point injections.

At press time, there are at least four treatments being tested for fibromyalgia, all vying to be the first drug approved by the FDA for treating fibromyalgia pain and stiffness. (One of these is interferon alpha (*Veldona*), an oral lozenge.) At this time, however, doctors may prescribe a variety of existing drugs to ease the many symptoms of the disease.

One of the main goals of doctors treating fibromyalgia is to promote deep, restorative sleep. The most effective drugs now available for this purpose are the tricyclic antidepressants. In addition, the use of another kind of antidepressant, selective serotonin reuptake inhibitors (SSRIs), might be taken along with tricyclics to boost energy. Fatigue is a common symptom of fibromyalgia also. Several other antidepressant medications may be used as part of fibromyalgia treatment. Some doctors may also prescribe benzodiazepines, a tranquilizer, to help fibromyalgia symptoms.

In addition, some people with fibromyalgia may find that the *anticonvulsant* medicine gabapentin (*Neurontin*) may ease leg pain,

tingling sensations or numbness that can be a symptom of fibromyalgia. See the section on anticonvulsants on p. 93.

**Common brands:** Antidepressants/tricyclics: amitryptiline hydrochloride (*Elavil, Endep*), doxepin (*Adapin, Sinequan*), nortriptyline (*Aventyl, Pamelor*)

Antidepressants/SSRIs: citalopram (*Celexa*), fluoxetine (*Prozac*), paroxetine (*Paxil*), setraline (*Zoloft*)

Other antidepressants: bupropion (*Wellbutrin, Zyban, Wellbutrin SR*), mirtazapime (*Remeron*), nefazodone (*Serzone*), trazodone (*Desyrel, Trazon, Trialodine*), venlafazine (*Effexor*).

Benzodiazepines: aprazolam (*Xanax*), clonazepam (*Klonopin*), lorazepam (*Ativan*), temazepam (*Restoril*), zaleplon (*Sonata*), zolpidem (*Ambien*)

Other Drugs: maprotiline (*Ludiomil*), trazodone (*Desyrel, Trazon, Trialodine*).

**Cautions:** For all tricyclic antidepressants, possible side effects can include constipation, dizziness, drowsiness, dry mouth, headache, tiredness and weight gain. There are numerous possible side effects for other types of antidepressants, including decrease in sexual desire or ability, drowsiness, anxiety or nervousness, dry mouth, gastrointestinal problems and more. Using alcohol along with many antidepressants can increase the effects of drowsiness or cause other problems. Ask your doctor or pharmacist for a complete list of side effects or cautions.

## Other Drugs

There are a number of other drugs that your doctor might prescribe for pain relief. Some of the most common are skeletal muscle relaxants, which we touched on briefly in the previous section. These drugs help to relax tensed, painful muscles in any part of the body. Doctors may prescribe them to treat conditions such as back or neck pain, temporomandibular joint disorder, fibromyalgia and more.

Muscle relaxants act in the central nervous system to send messages to the muscles to lessen their tension or spasm, which helps to relieve pain. Muscle relaxants also can make you feel sleepy or drowsy, which may be helpful if your pain has kept you from sleeping. These drugs should be used short-term, not as a long-term treatment.

**Common brands:** Carisoprodol (*Soma*), cyclobenzaprine (*Cycloflex, Flexeril*), orphenadrine (*Norflex*).

**Cautions:** Muscle relaxants can make you feel sleepy or drowsy, and this effect can be more intense if the drugs are taken by someone also using alcohol or taking central nervous system depressants (which include antihistamine drugs, prescription analgesics or narcotics, and sleeping medicines) or some tricyclic antidepressants. These drugs may cause blurred vision or clumsiness in some people, so use caution. It's probably best not to drive or operate any machinery while you are taking these drugs.

Tizanidine (*Zanaflex*) is an *antispastic* drug, or a drug that works in the central nervous system to relax muscles. Like the other muscle relaxants, tizanidine can ease painful muscle cramps, spasms and tension that may be caused by diseases like multiple sclerosis or spinal injuries. Similarly, it can cause drowsiness or lightheadedness that can be amplified if taken with central nervous system depressants or alcohol. It may also cause dryness of the mouth.

**Common brand:** Tizanidine (*Zanaflex*)

**Cautions:** Dizziness, sedation, liver damage (rare)

Gabapentin (*Neurontin*) is an anticonvulsant, or a drug used to fight seizures in people with epilepsy. But it's sometimes prescribed for other uses, including easing neuropathic pain. Neuropathic pain may be caused by actual damage to the nerves themselves or be related to diseases, like multiple sclerosis, diabetes or a painful skin condition called shingles, which is caused by the same virus that causes chickenpox. Some types of chronic back pain are neuropathic. While gabapentin usually doesn't have side effects, there is a risk of drowsiness, headache, fatigue, blurred vision, tremors (shaking of the limbs), anxiety or irregular eye movements in some people.

Central pain syndrome, which we learned about in Chapter One, is an extremely painful chronic condition that develops after damage to the central nervous system, such as after a stroke, injury or due to the disease multiple sclerosis. People with neuropathic pain often describe it as shooting, burning or stabbing. People with central pain syndrome often find some relief with gabapentin or nortriptyline.

**Common brand:** Gabapentin (*Neurontin*)

**Cautions:** Dizziness, drowsiness, headaches, loss of coordination, nausea

Other anticonvulsants that may be prescribed for jabbing-type pain are carbamazepine

(*Tegretol*) and phenytoin (*Dilantin*). Another drug that may be used for relief of pain is mexiletine (*Mexitil*), an antiarrythmic drug used to treat irregular heartbeats. Mexiletine may be used to relieve burning-type pain associated with neuropathic pain. Side effects of mexiletine may include dizziness, nausea, vomiting, difficulty walking or shaking hands. In a very small percentage of patients, a continuous infusion or intravenous application of an anesthetic such as lidocaine may be prescribed for chronic pain confined to a small area. Such an application might only take place in a pain center.

**Common brands:** Carbamazepine (*Tegretol, Atretol; Depitol; Epitol*)

**Cautions:** Upset stomach, drowsiness, vomiting, loss of appetite, diarrhea, hallucinations, insomnia, irritability, mental confusion, headache, dry mouth, speech problems, coordination problems, impotence, mouth and tongue irritation. Do not eat grapefruit or drink grapefruit juice one hour before or two hours after taking carbamazepine.

**Common brands:** Phenytoin (*Dilantin, Dilantin Infatabs, Dilantin Kapseals*)

**Cautions:** Upset stomach, drowsiness, redness, irritation, bleeding, swelling of the gums, vomiting, constipation, stomach pain, loss of taste, loss of appetite, weight loss, difficulty swallowing, mental confusion, blurred or double vision, insomnia, nervousness, muscle twitching, headache, increased hair growth

**Common brand:** Mexiletine (*Mexitil*)

**Cautions:** Dizziness, nausea, vomiting, difficulty walking or shaking hands

In the next chapter, we'll examine some other medical methods for treating pain, including some that involve surgical treatments and high-tech devices implanted in your body to offer continuous pain relief.

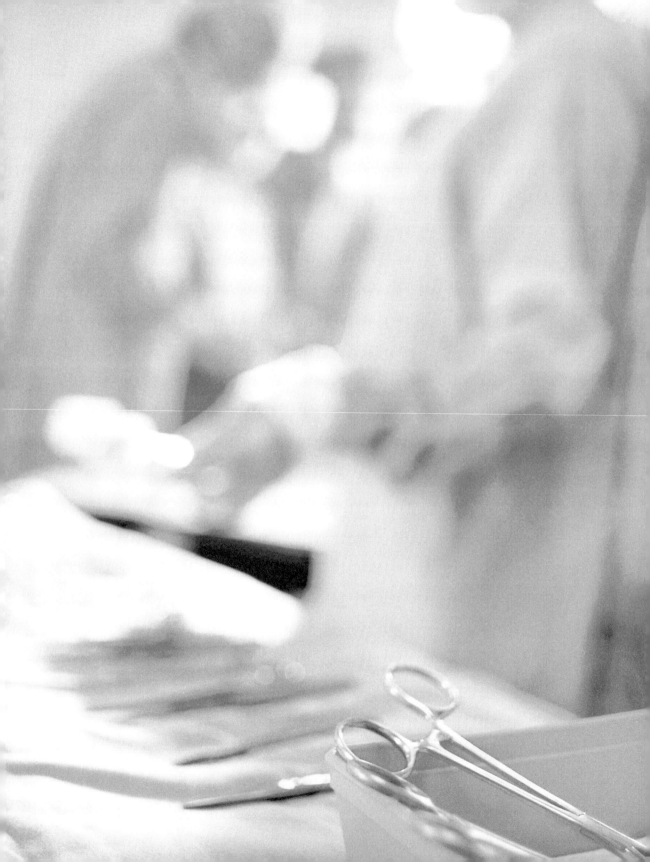

# Pumps, Implants, Surgery and More

6

# CHAPTER 6:
## PUMPS, IMPLANTS, SURGERY AND MORE

Chronic pain can interfere with every aspect of your life. When you are in constant pain, everything becomes difficult or impossible: work, recreation, sex, taking care of your family, household tasks, taking care of yourself. So finding the right pain-relief method is very important.

For many people, the medications discussed in the previous chapters – mostly taken by mouth in the form of pills – may not provide enough relief. In addition, these people may find that their primary-care physician runs out of solutions when it comes to their pain treatment, requiring a referral to a specialist or even to a pain center or clinic specializing in pain treatment. Whether or not you need to go to a pain clinic or pain center, your chronic pain may require treatment that goes beyond swallowing daily pills. Today's medicine offers some new methods of delivering pain medication and inflammation-fighting drugs to the source of your pain.

Hopefully, one of the many pain-relief medicines or techniques will work to help control your pain. Remember, using a multi-pronged approach – trying different medical, alternative and psychological methods as part of a comprehensive pain-management plan – may be the best way to deal with pain. By definition, chronic pain maybe constant, but with help, there's a good chance you can keep it under control so you can get on with your life.

## INJECTIONS AND IMPLANTS

The most common pain-relief treatments described in the previous two chapters are, primarily, taken in pill form. The medicine in these pills is digested in the stomach and absorbed into the bloodstream. There, it flows throughout the body and the active ingredients go to work. The medications address the malfunctioning body processes that are causing your pain, or limit the pain messages that travel from the site of your pain to your brain, where pain is perceived or "felt."

In some cases, it may be more effective to put a concentrated dose of medicine directly into the source of pain or injury – either a muscle, joint or nerve. Doctors do this by giving injections, or shots, or by placing implants within the body that release medication at a steady rate. Injections and implants may administer analgesics, anesthetic (or numbing) medicine, corticosteroids or a combination.

### Injections

Injections can send a high dose of medicine right to the affected area, delivering pain relief more quickly and directly. However, their effects may not last as long as those of oral medications (another term for pills that you swallow). For long-term pain relief or disease management, oral medications are preferable.

However, injections can provide additional pain relief for many people who have not found adequate relief through traditional drug treatments or non-drug therapies, such as heat or cold, or exercise. Injections may be *subcutaneous* (just under the skin); *intravenous* (directly into a vein); *epidural* or *intrathecal* (into a space around the spinal cord where pain receptor nerves are located); or *subdermal or intramuscular* (deeply into the skin or into a muscle). What type of pain you have or what type of pain injection treatment you are receiving determines the type of shot your doctor prefers in your case.

Doctors limit how many injections you can have for your pain, although this varies according to the medicine and the site of your pain. Too many injected corticosteroids, for example, might cause unpleasant side effects, making the treatment as difficult to bear as the pain. But many people prefer receiving an occasional injection to having surgery, so if injections can relieve pain until the need for surgery arises, they are beneficial.

Your doctor may perform aspiration of a joint, which means to use a syringe to drain fluid and other matter from the joint. For many types of arthritis, doctors remove fluid from the joint to examine so that they can determine the exact disease you have and treat it more effectively. If your doctor suspects you have gout, for example, he will probably remove some of the fluid from the affected joint to look for uric acid crystals that may be causing pain. Doctors also use needles to withdraw excess fluid from a swollen joint. This is a very common procedure. Removing excess fluid may help reduce swelling, and relieve pain and discomfort.

Injection therapy has relatively few side effects. However, some people do experience side effects from the medications injected, such as corticosteroids (see p. 82). Other complications include the risk of infection from the injection, a change in color of the skin around the injection, or problems associated with the medicine leaking into the surrounding tissue after it is injected.

There is also the risk that the doctor – usually a rheumatologist, orthopaedic surgeon, anesthesiologist, physiatrist (a doctor who supervises rehabilitation) or internist – may inject the needle in the wrong spot. This could cause a damaging puncture or rupture of a tendon, nerve, blood vessel or even the *dura mater,* the outer membrane covering the spinal cord. In some rare cases, nerves can be damaged due to an incorrectly placed injection.

## Joint Fluid Therapy

Some people with the chronic pain of knee osteoarthritis – a very common, often debilitating condition – get relief from joint fluid therapy. In osteoarthritis of the knee, some people experience a breakdown in production of the sticky, elastic fluid that helps cushion and protect the moving parts of the joint. When this happens, cartilage in the knee is unprotected and can deteriorate. When cartilage deteriorates, the person can experience painful, bone-on-bone rubbing when he moves the knee, such as in walking, bending or climbing stairs. This pain can be severe, making it difficult for the person to carry on normal activities.

Some people find relief through periodic injections of *hyaluronic acid*, which helps replenish the viscosity, or thickness and elasticity, of the joint fluid. This process is also called *viscosupplementation*. Joint fluid therapy may help reduce inflammation in the knee and also may help cartilage metabolism, or keep cartilage from breaking down so easily.

People with knee osteoarthritis who have not found pain relief from the standard treatments, such as NSAIDs, COX-2 drugs, analgesics, exercise or physical therapy, might try joint fluid therapy as another option. Joint fluid therapy injections are given by rheumatologists, orthopaedic surgeons (surgeons specializing in diseases or injuries of the bones) or primary-care physicians with experience in administering joint injections.

There are two different kinds of hyaluronic acid therapy approved by the Food and Drug Administration for the treatment of knee OA: sodium hyaluronate (*Hyalgan, Supartz*) and hylan G-F 20 (*Synvisc*). Doctors inject these fluids directly into the affected knee. If you use *Hyalgan,* your doctor will inject a series of three to five 2-milliliter (ml) weekly doses. If you use *Supartz*, your doctor will inject a series of five 2.5-ml doses administered weekly. *Synvisc* is given in a series of three 2-ml doses over a period of two weeks.

With any of these products, a local anesthetic, or numbing agent, may be applied to ease the pain or discomfort of the actual injection. In addition, your doctor may drain and remove fluid from the joint capsule to make room for the more viscous injected fluid, before injecting the hyaluronic acid.

Joint fluid therapy may relieve pain for a number of months. Doctors often suggest that people limit vigorous physical activity (such as sports or hiking) for one or two days after the injection.

Other than pain at the site of the injection, which may be relieved by giving an anesthetic first, joint fluid therapy carries few side effects. However, some people should not use these products. People with any allergic reactions to hyaluronan preparations, people who develop joint infections or skin infections at the site the injection, people with allergies to bird feathers, eggs and/or poultry should not use hyaluronic acid therapy.

## Corticosteroid Injections

While oral corticosteroids are a common treatment for the inflammation and pain of arthritis, doctors may also try a corticosteroid injection of the drug into the affected joint or joints. These injections sharply and quickly reduce your inflammation and pain. Yet when used over the long term, the effectiveness of injected corticosteroids can wane. They also can cause unpleasant or even dangerous side effects, including susceptibility to bruising; thinning of the bones or osteoporosis; weight gain; bloated face (sometimes called "moon face"); cataracts, which can cause vision loss or blindness; high blood pressure; and diabetes.

Research studies of injected corticosteroids into joints affected by osteoarthritis have shown mixed results. While some relief of symptoms was noted, the research also showed that the relief may be short-lived – only a few weeks – and that this treatment was perhaps only slightly more effective than *placebo,* or a "fake" injection. (See the box on the placebo effect, p. 117.) Some joints respond better than others to this type of injection treatment.

Corticosteroids are synthetic replicas of hormones that the body produces naturally, such as adrenaline or cortisol. By giving you higher doses of these hormones than your body would produce on its own, doctors hope to reduce inflammation. Commonly, doctors inject corticosteroids into the knee, hip, shoulder, elbow, and the facet or sacroiliac joints of the spine.

Sometimes, a local anesthetic drug is mixed in with the corticosteroid medicine for the injection. This anesthetic can provide almost immediate, temporary pain relief to the affected area as long as the doctor injects the spot accurately.

## Soft-Tissue Injections

As we have learned, soft tissues of the body, including muscles, bursae and tendons, can become inflamed and painful. Doctors can treat this type of inflammation with several types of injections, sending pain-relieving medicine straight to the source of the discomfort. There are two main types of soft-tissue injections: bursa injections and trigger point injections.

Bursa injections. Injection of corticosteroids is a direct treatment for the pain of bursitis, which can occur in any of the 150 bursae in your body. The most common sites of bursitis are the shoulder, hip, buttock and elbow. Bursae cushion the areas in the joints where bones meet muscles or tendons. When they become inflamed, moving the joint becomes very painful. Doctors can inject a dose of corticosteroids into the area to reduce the bursa inflammation, lessen the pain and restore mobility to the joint.

Trigger point injections. Also known as *field block injections*, trigger point injections refer to shots in the areas where muscles or *fascia,* fibrous tissues beneath your skin, are sensitive or painful. These injections may be helpful in cases of muscle pain or tension, or in fibromyalgia. Injecting a combination of anesthetic, to numb the area, and corticosteroid medication, to reduce inflammation and swelling, can provide pain relief and improve mobility in this area. Trigger point injections take between five and 15 minutes and may involve between one and five injections with a tiny needle. The treatment can take three to four days to take effect, but it can have long-term positive results in relieving pain.

## Nerve Block Injections

As we learned in Chapter One, you feel pain through your nerves. Nerve endings send pain messages through the spinal cord and into the brain, where you perceive them. Some injection treatments, called *nerve block injections,* can numb the nerve fibers around the damaged, diseased or painful area of the body so the nerve endings temporarily stop sending those pain messages.

Nerve block injections place a small amount of anesthetic medicine around the nerve fibers of the painful area. This relieves the pain for a short period of time, usually during a surgical procedure. For longer pain relief, doctors also can inject corticosteroids into the area around a nerve if there is swelling that is compressing the nerve and causing pain.

There are three main types of nerve block injections: peripheral, spinal and sympathetic.

- **Peripheral nerve blocks** are simply injections of anesthetic around the nerve to reduce sensation and pain. This type of nerve block injection might be done in smaller, concentrated areas of pain, such as in the ankle or elbow.
- **Spinal nerve blocks** are used for pain that affects wider areas of the body, such as your leg or back. In this type of nerve block, the doctor injects anesthetic medicine into or near the spinal column itself. You may have heard about *epidural injections,* one type of spinal nerve block that involves injecting anesthetic near the spinal column, but not directly into it. Epidurals are used to relieve severe pain in large areas of the body. Epidural blocks are used commonly in childbirth, making labor much easier on mothers. But now doctors are using epidural injections to relieve severe back pain, such as sciatica, a common and often debilitating problem. When doctors inject anesthetic directly into the spinal column,

the procedure is called intrathecal injection. This type of spinal nerve block may be used as anesthesia for major surgery also.

- **Sympathetic spinal nerve block injections** are another type of pain-relief injection that is used to control pain in the sympathetic nervous system. This system is a network of nerves that control basic life functions such as blood circulation, perspiration and body temperature. These nerves should control body functions without your awareness. People with the disease *reflex sympathetic dystrophy,* sometimes known as *complex regional pain syndrome,* may be experiencing pain due to damage or disruption in normal activity of these nerves. Doctors use sympathetic spinal nerve blocks to relieve pain from this type of disease, but controlled studies have not been performed to see if these blocks are really effective. Usually, doctors administer a series of sympathetic nerve blocks and monitor the patient's pain over time.

Injections of any type usually are given in the doctor's office or at a pain center, so you can be home and resting a few hours after your procedure. With any type of joint injection, doctors usually advise you to rest or limit your use of the joint from 24 to 48 hours after the injection. This rest period helps prevent leaking of the injected fluid, and also helps the medicine reduce the inflammation that may be causing pain. How long you may have to rest really depends on your situation. Your doctor will advise you.

## IMPLANTABLE DEVICES

Another relatively new option for people who do not get enough relief from traditional methods are implantable devices, tiny machines that pump prescribed amounts of medicine directly into the body to relieve pain. These devices are sometimes known as pumps or *intrathecal pain therapy*. This type of therapy is used for people with severe chronic pain or pain associated with nerve damage that does not respond to typical oral drugs.

*Neurostimulators* are another kind of implantable device that use electrical impulses instead of analgesics to block pain signals from reaching the brain. Neurostimulation often is used for people with nerve damage or neuropathic pain.

Both types of implants require you to have surgery and in many cases, a short hospital stay. The procedure to implant and activate the device lasts about one or two hours.

## Intrathecal Drug Delivery Pumps

Many people find pain relief through implanted drug pumps, and there are many benefits to using this type of drug delivery device. But how does it work?

Doctors must surgically implant a tiny pump that releases regular, small doses of analgesic medication (usually morphine or similar opioids) directly into the intrathecal space around the spinal cord. The intrathecal space is where pain messages are most effectively interrupted. Through a catheter, a slender, flexible delivery tube, the pump delivers the medicine to this space. The pump is set by your doctor to release medicine at a particular interval (the dose depends on your level of pain).

Because the spinal cord is the body's telephone line for pain messages, blocking or interrupting the transmission of the messages helps relieve pain. The pump device usually is inserted through an incision in the lower abdomen, or near where your belt sits on your body.

Implantable pain-relief devices involve risks and it's very important to place the device properly. Usually, doctors perform a test or trial run of the implant using a temporary catheter attached to a pump that is outside your body. This test typically lasts for about three days. This trial run allows you and your doctor to see how effective the treatment will be, and how much your abilities to move around or perform daily tasks improve.

For people with severe, chronic pain, these devices can be very effective for a number of reasons, not the least of which is convenience. The pumps release medicine automatically into the body, which means you don't have to remember to take pills on a schedule. In addition, the devices release the drug at regular intervals, giving a continuous stream of pain-relieving medication to the person in pain.

In addition, some people experience fewer side effects, such as nausea or grogginess, from implantable devices than from taking pills. In addition, intrathecal pumps often can relieve pain with much lower doses of medicine than a person taking analgesics in pill form would require.

There are risks to any kind of treatment. Implants or pumps, because they involve surgery, do carry risks. These risks include allergic reactions to the medicine, bleeding, problems with the device or improper implantation, headaches, injuries to the spinal cord, paralysis or infections from the implantation. The devices may leak or shift, or even fail to work, requiring additional surgery. (If the device fails to release the drug as prescribed, you could experience an overdose of the drug, so this is a strong concern.) People with implantable devices must see their doctor regularly to refill the medicine in the pump and to make sure it is running properly.

## Neurostimulation Devices

Another useful type of implanted device uses electricity, rather than analgesic drugs, to relieve pain. This technique, called *spinal cord stimulation* or *implanted neurostimulation*, involves delivery of electrical impulses through a tiny, carefully placed wire inside the body. The impulses stimulate the nerves on the spinal cord to interrupt the pain signal transmission.

Like intrathecal pain therapy, neurostimulation involves surgery. A surgeon will implant a tiny device, called a lead, near your spinal cord or peripheral nerve. The lead is a special, flexible, insulated wire designed for medical use. The lead and another small device called a neurostimulator send electrical impulses to the spinal cord to block pain signals from reaching the brain.

The neurostimulator is powered either by an implanted battery (known as a fully implanted neurostimulation system) or an external power source (known as a radio frequency system).

With the fully implanted system, the battery power source and all the wiring is inside your body. With the external power source, you will have a small antenna attached to your skin with adhesive, and you must carry a battery pack, which looks like a small TV remote control or personal pager.

With neurostimulation therapy, you may feel the impulses as a tingling sensation. Some people compare this sensation to when you rub your elbow or "funny bone" after bumping it – the rubbing helps to mask and soothe the sudden pain you feel.

Another type of neurostimulation method is peripheral nerve stimulation, in which the surgeon places the lead near the specific peripheral nerve that is damaged and causing pain. (See p. 9 for more on the peripheral nerves.) Peripheral nerve stimulation uses only the external radio frequency system for power.

As with intrathecal pumps, most doctors require a trial run of a neurostimulation device. This trial period usually lasts a few days. You and your doctor will test and monitor your response to the device. If it works properly and you do notice benefit, you'll undergo a short operation to implant the device, followed by a brief hospital stay.

If neurostimulation seems like an option you might be interested in, it's important to talk to your doctor about the risks and cautions. The impulses may be uncomfortable, feeling like electrical shocks or jolts. Some people have an allergic reaction to the device or develop an infection related to the surgery. Serious reactions, like a *hematoma* (a swollen collection of blood, almost like a blood-filled sac) or paralysis, are rare, but could occur. Because these devices are very expensive, insurance coverage should be investigated.

Because you have an electronic implant in your body, outside electronic devices like power tools or airport security scanners might interfere with your neurostimulator. You should ask your doctor about any risks and what precautions you should take to prevent problems. There may be some activities you should avoid while using your neurostimulator, or you should at least be prepared for what reactions you may experience. Your doctor may be able to adjust the power of your neurostimulator if you notice unpleasant jolts or sensations often due to outside electrical stimulation.

## SURGICAL PAIN-RELIEF PROCEDURES

People with serious chronic pain may exhaust other options for pain relief, such as drugs or alternative therapies, and find that surgery is the next best step. Surgery can be a beneficial but serious treatment for extreme chronic pain.

Many people with arthritis have joint surgery, such as arthroplasty or total joint replacements, as a way to remove damaged, painful joints and restore mobility. In other cases, surgeons can treat neuropathic pain through implantation devices or specific nerve surgeries designed to treat the source of severe pain. Joint and bone surgeries are performed by orthopaedic surgeons, while nerve surgeries are performed by specialists called neurosurgeons.

All of these procedures require major surgery, a hospital stay, lengthy recovery and rehabilitation, and often, significant cost (this may be covered by your insurance).

Some surgical procedures produce amazing results. A person with a severely damaged joint due to osteoarthritis or rheumatoid arthritis can find, after joint replacement surgery and recovery, that their pain is reduced and their mobility is greatly restored. Other people find that surgery is not as effective, or serves as a partial treatment for their serious pain.

Some of the most common forms of surgery used to treat arthritis pain are outlined in the following sections.

## Arthroplasty or Total Joint Replacement

Arthroplasty, or total joint replacement, involves removing damaged joints and replacing them with a new joint component made of metal, ceramic and plastic. Hundreds of thousands of joints are replaced annually, including hips, knees, shoulders, elbows, fingers and knuckles.

The surgeon secures the new, artificial joint with either special bone cement or through a cementless procedure where the body's tissues and bone grow slowly around the joint to hold it in place. Arthroplasty requires weeks of recovery and rehabilitation. Some new surgical techniques for joint replacements are less invasive, requiring a smaller incision and shorter recovery time after surgery. In addition, there are new, higher-flexibility knee replacements that allow greater range of motion for the knee after surgery. Not everyone may qualify for these new procedures; ask your doctor for more information or to see if he is trained in these types of procedures.

## Arthroscopy

Arthroscopy (see p. 40) is widely practiced as a diagnostic surgery to determine the cause of the pain. Some surgeons use arthroscopy to perform many different surgical procedures without having to make a large incision in the body. Making a smaller incision and using an arthroscope can make surgery and recovery much easier.

Some surgeons also may use arthroscopy to treat minor damage to cartilage, bones, ligaments or tendons that may be causing pain. Arthroscopy procedures are most often done on knees and shoulders. Doctors would use the arthroscope to view small damage to joints, and then trim ragged cartilage or remove loose bits of tissue that may be causing discomfort or pain. A recent study questioned the efficacy or necessity of such a procedure, but some surgeons may use it.

## Other Common Surgeries

Osteotomy. Osteotomy is the cutting and reshaping of bone that may be out of alignment due to arthritis, causing pain and impaired movement. Osteotomy may correct the way the bones of the joint fit together, particularly for hips and knees.

Arthrodesis. In arthrodesis, a surgeon cuts the bones of the arthritis-damaged joint and fuses the ends of the bones together, holding them with a pin or rod that is inserted into the bones. This procedure creates a more stable, but rather immobile, joint. However, it may allow a person with severe arthritis to reduce pain and increase ability to move around, if not to bend the joint as he once could.

Resection. In resection surgery, the surgeon removes a damaged portion of the bones in a joint, leaving a small space between the joint and various soft tissues. Scar tissue fills the space, allowing more flexibility than before, but less stability.

Synovectomy. In synovectomy, a surgeon removes damaged or inflamed parts of the synovium, or joint lining (which can become inflamed and painful in some forms of arthritis). Sometimes, a surgeon can perform a synovectomy using an arthroscope, requiring a less invasive operation and shorter recovery time. Synovectomy is not always a permanent solution: Sometimes the synovium grows back, only to flare up in pain again.

For more information on many types of joint surgery, read *All You Need To Know About Joint Surgery: Preparing for Surgery, Recovery and an Active New Lifestyle*. Published by the Arthritis Foundation, this comprehensive book covers the most common types of joint surgery, explains the procedures, and prepares you for surgery, recovery and rehabilitation. It's available by calling (800) 207-8633 or online at www.arthritis.org.

## Nerve-Related Surgeries

For neuropathic or nerve-related pain, neuro-surgeons can perform different operations to treat the pain at its source: the damaged or inflamed nerves. We have already learned about nerve blocks, but here are a few more of the most common procedures to treat neuro-pathic pain:

- **Neurectomy** (including peripheral neurec-tomy) is a procedure to remove the dam-aged peripheral nerve that is causing pain.
- In **spinal dorsal rhizotomy**, usually reserved for severe chronic pain or even cancer-related pain, the surgeon carefully cuts the roots of one or more of the dam-aged nerves that radiates from the spine, or the nerve root where a painful condition is occurring. Other rhizotomy procedures include cranial rhizotomy, selective rhizo-tomy and trigeminal rhizotomy.
- **Sympathectomy** or **sympathetic blockade** describes a procedure in which the surgeon injects a drug, usually guanethidine, to eliminate pain in a specific area, such as an arm or leg. People with heart-related pain, vasculitis, reflex sympathetic dystrophy syn-drome or other conditions may undergo this procedure.
- **Deep brain stimulation or intracerebral stimulation** is a very new form of internal nerve treatment involving surgical stimula-tion of the thalamus portion of the brain. This treatment usually is reserved for peo-ple with serious neuropathic pain, such as central pain syndrome.

With any pain-relieving medications or devices, there are side effects, risks and cau-tions. In addition, some people may find that the drug or device may simply fail to relieve their pain. In these cases, doctors sometimes say this person has *intractable pain,* meaning that their pain has not responded to any treat-ment available. If you do find that you have intractable pain, there may be other options for finding relief: alternative or complemen-tary therapies. We'll discuss these therapies in the next chapter.

Even if drugs or devices do provide some pain relief, you may find that incorporating alternative therapies and lifestyle changes (such as adopting an exercise plan or chang-ing your diet) can help you better manage your pain and overall health. In addition, they may help you cope better with your chronic pain and the disease that causes it.

For people with chronic pain, developing a plan for coping is essential. Some pain cen-ters offer guidance in coping with chronic pain, so if there is a center in your area (see www.asahq.org, the American Society of Anes-thesiologists, to learn more), consider taking advantage of its services.

The Arthritis Foundation also has a pro-gram available through its more than 150 chapter and branch offices nationwide called *Speaking of Pain.* This program, led by trained volunteers, discusses chronic pain manage-ment and offers practical strategies for coping with chronic pain. To find an Arthritis Foun-dation office near you, call (800) 283-7800 or log on to www.arthritis.org.

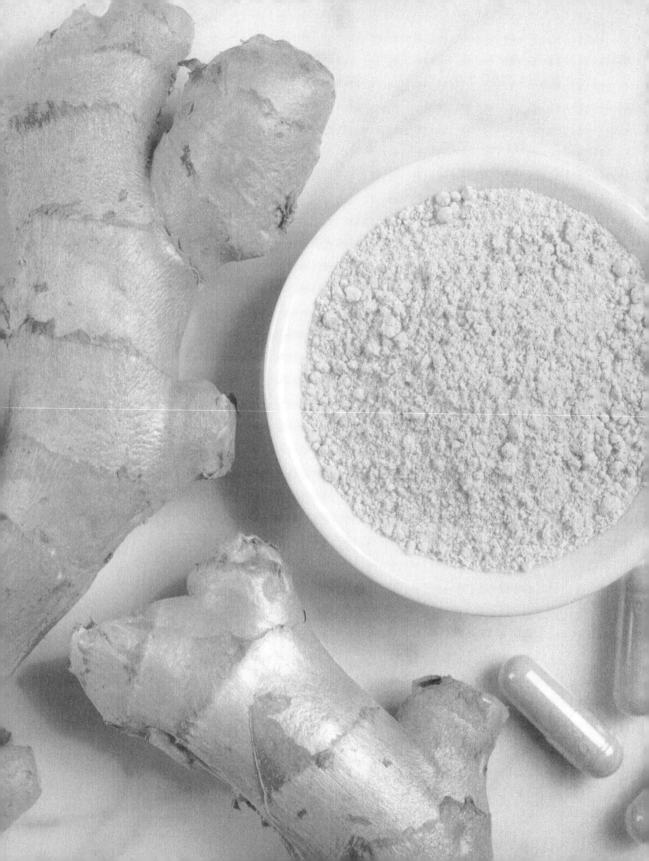

# Natural Options:
# Herbs, Supplements
# and More

7

# CHAPTER 7: NATURAL OPTIONS: HERBS, SUPPLEMENTS AND MORE

Most people with chronic pain wish they could find relief in a simple pill. But for most people with arthritis, fibromyalgia, chronic back problems or other painful conditions, controlling pain on a daily basis means trying a variety of techniques and strategies.

These strategies can include drugs, lifestyle or habit changes, and alternative therapies as part of the pain-management plan that you create with your doctor's supervision. With your doctor's help, you can identify what therapies are most effective for you and what therapies to avoid.

If you have chronic pain, you've probably read magazine articles or heard friends talk about alternative therapies. Also called *complementary* therapies or *natural medicine*, this category of treatments contains many different types of pain-relief options. Some alternatives involve the help of a *practitioner* or professional trained or skilled in administering these therapies. Other strategies are things you may try on your own.

There are some controversies associated with alternative therapies and their use. There are few studies to support the efficacy of most of these therapies. Yet some are probably quite beneficial for pain relief. The best source of information and advice is your doctor. Your doctor will be able to discuss alternative options for pain relief and steer you toward treatments that are more likely to work.

Let's learn more about the differences between alternative and medical treatments, and why some treatments may fall somewhere between the lines.

## WHAT IS AN ALTERNATIVE THERAPY?

Alternative therapy is a loose, umbrella term for a group of treatments that fall outside the standard medical therapies prescribed by doctors. Medical therapies include drugs, surgery, physical therapy, occupational therapy and any treatment supervised by a medical doctor or physical or occupational therapist. Whatever is left – and this category includes a wide variety of treatments – may be considered alternative.

While some therapies may not fall so easily into one category or the other, we'll try to discuss the many pain-relief therapies in two main classifications: medical and alternative. For purposes of this discussion, medical treatments include drugs, implanted devices and surgery, or anything prescribed or regulated by a medical professional such as a doctor or physical therapist. Alternative treatments include just about everything else, including treatments performed or suggested by a practitioner such as a chiropractor.

The terminology can be confusing. Some people call therapies like acupuncture or herbal supplements "traditional medicine" because people have been using these therapies for centuries. Yet we now refer to drugs and surgery as "traditional medicine" and call herbs, acupuncture or other non-medical treatments "alternative."

While some medical doctors once ignored alternative therapies as either bogus or inadvisable, many doctors now accept their use by patients and discuss these treatments as part of an overall pain-management plan. Some doctors even practice *integrative medicine,* a blend of mainstream medical treatments and alternative or natural therapies.

Many people consider alternative therapies safer because they are more "natural." Yet many of these treatments have side effects or risks. Some natural treatments contain the same basic ingredient as many drugs, so if you take an herbal supplement and a drug that do the same thing, you may be getting too much medicine at once.

The line between drugs and natural treatments is not so clear. In fact, the first drugs for treating pain came from natural sources, such as opium poppies (narcotic analgesics), willow tree bark (aspirin and other salicylate NSAIDs) and others. For centuries, physicians offered their patients these preparations to relieve pain and other symptoms. Over time, scientists refined these substances or discovered ways to make them more effective. Even now, scientists work constantly to make drugs safer and more effective. Many drugs are synthetic versions of chemicals your body produces naturally, like hormones. The synthetic versions are designed to work more effectively than the natural versions. But they are often the same chemical.

Still, some people feel uncomfortable using a lot of drugs to treat their pain. They believe that taking a lot of "chemicals" is "unnatural" and not as healthy as using treatments that seem closer to their natural state. Some people may be frustrated by the lack of pain relief offered by their drugs, so they turn to alternative treatments in the hope that they will be more effective. Alternative treatments, like over-the-counter drugs, don't require a prescription, so a person in pain can just go to the store, read labels and buy whatever they want to try. While this seems easier than going to your doctor, it can also be a dangerous game.

No matter what alternative therapy you try, it's very important first to discuss what you want to use with your doctor. These "natural therapies" can be very powerful medicines or treatments. They may interfere with the drugs your doctor has prescribed. So talk to your doctor about alternative therapies. He may be able to suggest alternative treatments that will be effective for relieving your pain. He also will help you avoid those therapies that will interfere with your current medications or those that don't work at all.

## What's the Controversy About Alternatives?

In the past, many medical doctors were skeptical of alternative therapies. These therapies were untested by scientists or the Food and Drug Administration (FDA), the federal agency that regulates and approves drugs. If you wished to try any alternative treatment, you did so at your own risk and without any guidance or approval from your doctor, pharmacist or even reputable organizations and government agencies that regulate health treatments.

These days, more and more Americans are using alternative treatments and purchasing products and services that fall into this category. This trend has awakened many established government and medical institutions. They are beginning to look more closely and seriously at alternative and complementary therapies. Respected universities and medical research institutions now conduct scientific studies on these therapies to see if they are safe and effective for patients to use.

In the late 1990s, the National Institutes of Health formed the National Center for Complementary and Alternative Medicine (NCCAM), an agency designed to study the many alternative medical therapies on the market. Recently, the NCCAM and 16 co-sponsors from the federal government announced the launch of a major study of the scientific and policy implications of the use of complementary and alternative medicine by Americans. This study, which will take nearly two years to complete at a cost of $1 million, is conducted by the Institute of Medicine, a private, not-for-profit, non-governmental institution chartered by the U.S. Congress. Experts in medical research will serve as volunteer panelists for the study.

Despite these and other major studies, there is still so much we do not know about alternative and complementary therapies. Alternative therapies are still not approved by the FDA, so when you use them, you do so at your own risk. By talking to your doctor and/or pharmacist before trying an alternative treatment, you can at least get the professional opinion of someone you know and trust before trying something new. When you're in pain, you may be willing to try anything in the hopes of finding relief. But you don't want to try something that will do more harm than good, and you don't want to waste your time and money on treatments that may do nothing at all.

Drugs and other medical treatments go through a very serious, lengthy process of testing and retesting to determine their effectiveness and possible risks of their use. Once the FDA approves medications, doctors may prescribe them, but even then, continued studies and examinations track any possible problems associated with the drugs' use.

Some alternative therapies have undergone scientific, controlled studies by reputable institutions such as universities, but many have not undergone any scientific study at all. No approval from the FDA is necessary for them to be sold to the public. In addition, companies can market these products as pain relievers. This regulatory loophole allows many treatments to be marketed and sold to the public without any evidence that they work to relieve pain. There are thousands of pain-relief products sold through magazines, TV infomercials, Internet ads, health-food stores and word of mouth, but many probably don't work at all. In this chapter, we'll discuss some unproven remedies and some treatments that probably don't do anything to relieve your pain.

# Alternatives: Be Savvy

If you are in pain, you may be willing to try anything to find relief. You will see hundreds of magazine ads, infomercials and Internet banner ads that tout various products or devices for pain relief. You may hear your friends talk about amazing new treatments that work better than drugs with no side effects. You may pick up bottles of herbal supplements at the supermarket, pharmacy or health-food store with labels that claim astonishing pain relief and restoration of mobility, strength and energy – all available to you by taking a simple pill.

If you're considering any complementary or alternative treatment, do your homework first. Don't assume a product is safe just because the label or advertising says it's "natural." Remember: Hemlock, the deadly poison, is natural, too.

Here are some useful guidelines to follow as you consider alternative or complementary treatments:

- **Know the facts about the therapy.** Although drugs and other medical treatments are monitored and regulated by the U.S. government (through agencies like the FDA), alternative therapies do not have to undergo that type of scrutiny to be marketed to the public. This is a very important loophole in the system. You may have to conduct some of your own research about the treatment, or ask your doctor or pharmacist.

- **Buyer beware.** If the packaging or advertising of a product or a practitioner of a therapy makes unrealistic pain-relief claims, such as, "It will cure your disease for good," be wary of this product. If a practitioner (such as an acupuncturist or chiropractor) suggests you discontinue your conventional medical treatments, consider it a strong warning that something is not right. Most reputable practitioners try to work in conjunction with your medical treatment, understanding that their therapy is just one part of your total pain-management plan.

- **Do your own research.** Read up on any alternative therapies you wish to try. Many books and Web sites are devoted to topics related to alternative therapies. Ask your doctor to provide any knowledge he has about the treatment. Two good sources of information about common alternative treatments are the *Arthritis Foundation's Guide to Alternative Therapies*, available by calling (800) 207-8633, by visiting www.arthritis.org, or at bookstores; and the NCCAM. The NCCAM offers a free packet of information on alternative therapies. Request this packet by writing to the NCCAM Clearinghouse, P.O. Box 8218, Silver Spring, MD 20807-8218.

# Alternatives: Be Savvy

- **Search the Internet.** There are numerous Web sites devoted to information about alternative and complementary therapies for chronic pain and other conditions. However, some may provide unsubstantiated information, some may exist mainly to sell you products and some may be biased toward a particular health philosophy. You will have to use your own judgment about the validity of the information you collect online. The Arthritis Foundation Web site, www.arthritis.org, offers some information about alternative therapies for treating chronic pain. In addition, here are a few useful, reputable sites to explore:

The National Center for Complementary and Alternative
  Medicine: www.nccam.nih.gov

The American Society of Anesthesiologists: www.asahq.org

The Richard and Hinda Rosenthal Center for Complementary and Alternative
  Medicine at Columbia University: www.rosenthal.hs.columbia.edu

WebMD: www.webmd.com

Alternative Medicine magazine: www.alternativemedicine.com

- **Be a healthy skeptic.** Just as you would be skeptical when buying a gadget for your car or your home, be skeptical where your health is concerned. Avoid treatments that claim to work by a secret formula, or be a magical cure or miraculous breakthrough. Scientists work very hard to find miraculous breakthroughs for pain relief.

While important treatments may be found in nature or outside the laboratory, if they really work well, chances are they won't be secret for long! Be wary of products that are only advertised in the backs of magazines, through phone marketing or through direct mail. Reputable treatments will be reported in medical journals and picked up by the mainstream press. How manufacturers verify the product's claims is important as well – if the product only has testimonials as proof that it works, rather than scientific studies, be wary.

- **Talk openly with your doctor.** Tell your doctor about any treatment you use, whether alternative, conventional or over-the-counter. Your doctor knows a great deal about the many pain-relief treatments available. He can talk to you about possible side effects and negative interactions with drugs you may be taking. Your doctor should work with you to oversee your pain-management plan and decide what new therapies are of possible benefit.

- **Watch out for high price tags.** Some alternative treatments can be expensive and they probably won't be covered by your insurance policy. Read your policy carefully to learn what's covered and under what circumstances. Some policies do allow for certain types of alternative treatment, such as chiropractic adjustments or acupuncture, but may not cover supplements. Compare the costs of various treatments and decide what options offer the most pain-relief bang for the buck.

- **Find a reputable practitioner.** If you do use an alternative treatment that requires a practitioner, seek out a qualified professional. Some state boards or national associations license practitioners of particular therapies. Find out about professional societies that provide certification for these treatments and ask for a referral list.

- **Don't ditch something that does the job already.** If you do try an alternative treatment for pain, don't stop taking your prescribed drugs. This could cause problems or interrupt your pain relief. Talk to your doctor to make sure this treatment is safe to use with your prescribed drugs, or ask him if you might temporarily stop or reduce your medication to try an alternative treatment instead.

- **Don't mix and match.** Be cautious about potential interactions between your drugs, both prescription and over-the-counter, and any herbal medicines or treatments you try. Ask your doctor or pharmacist before adding any natural or herbal treatment to your pain-management plan. Even something that seems harmless may affect the way your prescribed treatments work.

In recent years, the United States government and the medical establishment have taken alternative therapies more seriously, and scientists are beginning to study alternative therapies for effectiveness and safety. Still, there is no governmental regulation of these therapies, so it's important for you to be a wise consumer when experimenting. The guidelines in this chapter offer some steps you may wish to take to find the most effective treatments.

One big risk associated with trying alternative treatments without a doctor's advice is that you may not be getting what you paid for. Because herbs, nutritional supplements and other natural remedies available in drugstores, health-food stores and supermarkets are not regulated by the FDA, nor required to undergo the agency's rigorous approval process, there's no guarantee the remedy will be effective or safe despite label claims. There is no guarantee that the remedy contains the ingredients or the amount of the ingredient listed on the label. You could be wasting your time, money and patience.

If you do purchase herbs, supplements or natural remedies, ask your doctor or pharmacist to recommend particular brands that are more reputable. Don't rely on the advice of friends or unqualified, unlicensed staff in health-food stores.

## HERBS AND SUPPLEMENTS FOR CHRONIC PAIN

When most people think of alternative therapies, they think of herbs, vitamins and supplements, also known as nutritional or natural supplements. These items seem very much like drugs. They often come in pill, capsule, liquid or ointment form and are sold in many drugstores. Most people have good feelings about taking vitamins, herbs, minerals or natural-based compounds, because using something "natural" suggests promotion of good health.

In the past, these items (other than vitamins and minerals) were only found in health-food stores or sold through mail-order catalogs. But supplements are now available in almost every pharmacy, supermarket and discount department store. They are advertised everywhere, promoted and sold over the Internet and through direct-marketing networks. Some doctors may offer samples or coupons for the products to patients in their offices.

More and more studies are being conducted on herbs, vitamins and supplements to determine their *efficacy* (whether or not they actually work) and safety for humans. There are different types of studies performed on drugs as well as supplements. Studies performed in a laboratory are known as *in vitro* (Latin for "in glass," as in a test tube), and studies performed on animals or humans are known as *in vivo* (Latin for "in life"). Reliable scientific studies should be performed under controlled circumstances. In other words, two groups of people selected according to specific qualifications (such as their age, disease, level of pain) should be tested. One group would receive the supplement to be tested, and the other group would receive a placebo, or fake supplement. (See the box on p. 117 about the "placebo effect.") The most reliable tests are "blind" studies, where no

# THE PLACEBO EFFECT

Scientists often test drugs, supplements and other treatments to see if they really work. The most reliable studies use a group of people to test the treatment, where half receive the actual treatment and the other half receive a phony version of the treatment, called a *placebo*. (Placebo (plah-*see*-bo) is a Latin word meaning "I will please.")

No participants in a study should know whether or not they received the actual treatment or the placebo. Why? By doing this, researchers learn if the people who use the treatment are really gaining some benefit from it. If the group who takes the real treatment sees the same benefit as the group who takes the placebo or phony treatment, then the treatment may be ineffective.

How could the people who took a placebo – something like a capsule filled with sugar – gain any pain-relief benefit? There is a strange phenomenon called the placebo effect at work. Scientists have observed that some people sense improvement in their symptoms just because they take a treatment that they think they will benefit from. This inexplicable improvement in symptoms may be due to the power of the mind or suggestion. People believe that the pill (which may be no more than a piece of candy disguised to look like a pill) will help them because pills containing real medicine often do. They associate pills, especially pills given to them by a doctor, nurse or other official-looking health-care professional, as helpful. Their belief that the pill will help their pain is so strong that they begin to feel relief. Studies have shown that as many as 30 to 35 percent of people receiving placebos report some initial relief from symptoms. However, pain usually returns for most of these people.

That doesn't mean that we should toss out all of our prescription medicines and just eat candy corn. The placebo effect has to do with the power of the mind to heal, and that's very important and real. Using your mind to help you cope with symptoms and even reduce your sensation of pain is a good strategy that we will discuss more in Chapter Eight. But most people who sense improvement from a placebo in a trial will probably start feeling their pain again soon. That's because they haven't taken anything for the pain that will really address the physical process behind the pain. Researchers continue to study the placebo effect in an attempt to understand the power of the mind to affect healing and pain relief.

participants know whether they are receiving the real treatment or the placebo.

As we will learn in this chapter, we don't have a great deal of scientific data to say whether or not most of these supplements work. Many have possible side effects or cautions associated with their use, and you and your doctor should discuss whether you should try them or not. In many cases, it may be safe to use these supplements as part of your pain-management plan, but there's no guarantee they will work. It could be a "may not help, but can't really hurt" situation, so the decision to use them or not is up to you.

Almost half of Americans report having used some type of dietary or nutritional supplement in the recent past. Because supplements are widely available and easy to use, it's no wonder they are so popular for people seeking pain relief.

However, there are still some concerns. Do these supplements do what they claim to do? Are they safe to use? For the latest information on many common supplements used for chronic pain relief, contact the Arthritis Foundation to request *Arthritis Today's Supplement Guide,* available by calling (800) 283-7800 or logging onto www.arthritis.org.

Here are some commonly used supplements for treating chronic pain, fatigue and inflammation.

## Glucosamine and Chondroitin Sulfate

If you have arthritis or any type of joint pain, you've probably heard of glucosamine and chondroitin sulfate. The market is full of different brands of these popular supplements, and the media has covered the strong reports of their effectiveness in the news.

Both glucosamine and chondroitin sulfate come in various forms depending on the preparation and brand: capsules, tablets, liquid or powder. Glucosamine (also known as glucosamine sulfate) is made from the shells of crustaceans (shrimp, lobster and/or crab), and chondroitin sulfate is made from the tracheas (windpipes) of cattle or pork byproducts. Both products may be, in the supplement form, made from animal products, but they are similar to the material that makes up human cartilage.

Chondroitin sulfate is also found in human bone and tendon. Cartilage is the rubbery, flexible material in the body that allows you to move your joints freely and comfortably. Cartilage cushions bones where they meet at joints.

When people develop arthritis or many arthritis-related diseases, their cartilage often deteriorates. It is believed that supplements like glucosamine and chondroitin sulfate help to repair or restore that cartilage, easing movement and reducing pain. These supplements may relieve pain in people with osteoarthritis on a similar scale with NSAIDs, although they may take twice as long to take effect.

Glucosamine supposedly helps the body grow, repair or retain cartilage in the body's joints. It also helps cartilage absorb water, lubricating the joint so it moves more easily. Studies on glucosamine have been promising; two recent studies found that the supplement did relieve pain and improve movement function.

Chondroitin is believed to reduce pain and improve joint function by helping collagen (the main component of cartilage) absorb the impact of joint movement better. It's also supposed to block the deteriorating action of certain enzymes (body chemicals that can be corrosive in some instances) in the body that may break down cartilage. But there is no current proof that chondroitin stops or reverses the loss of cartilage in the body, as some users believe.

Studies of glucosamine have been more scientific and conclusive than those of chondroitin. The NIH is now conducting a major study on both supplements (in addition to a combination mixture) in people with knee osteoarthritis; results are expected in 2005. Some products combine glucosamine and chondroitin sulfate, but no studies show that this combination is more effective than taking either supplement on its own.

**Possible cautions or side effects of chondroitin:** diarrhea, constipation and abdominal pain. People who also take blood-thinning medications like NSAIDs might see an increased risk of bleeding if they also take chondroitin. Chondroitin sulfate supplements often come from cow trachea, so there is some concern that supplements may come from cattle infected with mad cow disease, a serious illness common in livestock in Europe in recent years.

**Possible cautions or side effects of glucosamine:** Mild stomach upset, nausea, heartburn, diarrhea, constipation, increased blood pressure and increased blood glucose, cholesterol and triglyceride levels. If you have diabetes, talk to your doctor before trying glucosamine. If you are allergic to shellfish, avoid using glucosamine as these supplements are made from their shells.

## Boswellia

Boswellia, also known as Indian frankincense, frankincense or salai guggal, is a supplement derived from the bark of the Boswellia tree found in India, North Africa and parts of the Middle East. Boswellia comes in capsule or pill form, and the supplement supposedly reduces inflammation and treats various symptoms of painful diseases like osteoarthritis, rheumatoid arthritis and bursitis.

Few clinical studies have been performed on boswellia, but some studies show that the supplement may inhibit leukotriene synthesis, which contributes to inflammation. But studies have failed to consistently show any relief from pain and inflammation.

**Possible side effects:** Diarrhea, nausea or rash.

## Bromelain

Made from pineapples, bromelain is an enzyme in the tropical fruit's juice that breaks down protein. It's available in tablet form. Bromelain is meant to decrease pain in arthritis and increase joint mobility.

Some evidence supports the claim that bromelain and other protein-dissolving enzymes can relieve pain and inflammation much as

NSAIDs do. And bromelain is probably quite safe to use. One in vivo study on humans showed that a bromelain supplement containing the enzymes rutin and trypsin relieved pain in 73 people with knee osteoarthritis, an effect similar to taking an NSAID. Studies at this time don't show that taking bromelain alone will relieve arthritis pain effectively, but it may be a good supplement to your overall pain-management plan. In addition, bromelain may help reduce swelling after surgery or injury, which may decrease discomfort.

**Possible side effects:** Stomach upset and diarrhea. Bromelain may increase the effect of blood-thinning medicines.

## Cat's Claw

Cat's claw is a supplement made from the dried root bark of a wild vine found in the Amazon region of Peru. The vine's claw-shaped thorns give the supplement its name. It's sold in capsule, tablet or tea bag (which must be steeped in hot water) form.

Centuries ago, cat's claw vine was used a treatment for inflammation and pain in bones or joints, and some people with knee osteoarthritis use the supplement to reduce inflammation and pain. At least one in vivo study performed on animals shows that cat's claw may prevent inflammation and other cell damage. Another study showed that freeze-dried cat's claw prevented knee pain in people with osteoarthritis.

**Possible side effects:** Headache, dizziness and vomiting. Cat's claw may also lower blood pressure and adversely affect people with autoimmune disorders, so people with rheumatoid arthritis, lupus or multiple sclerosis should not use it.

## Cetyl Myristoleate (CMO)

CMO comes from a waxy, fatlike substance found in mice. Available in pill or cream form, it's also known as cetyl-M. This substance is believed to prevent mice from getting arthritis.

CMO is advertised widely as a fast-acting cure for many forms of arthritis, but there is no scientific evidence at this time that these claims are true. CMO's claims stem from a 1993 study showing that CMO injections prevented arthritis in rats. However, no evidence exists that the substance that keeps rodents from getting arthritis will work in humans. CMO's claims include lubricating joints, regulating the immune system, easing inflammation, and reducing painful symptoms of many arthritis-related diseases.

One study on rats isn't reason enough to try a supplement that could be dangerous in people. Perhaps the most dangerous aspect of CMO is that some CMO vendors advise people considering the supplement to stop taking methotrexate and corticosteroids first (explaining that these drugs could interfere with CMO's action). As we noted previously, this practice is very dangerous. Your prescribed drugs have scientific studies behind them to prove their efficacy and are regulated by the FDA. People with rheumatoid arthritis who stop taking their drugs to try CMO may wind up with irreparable joint damage and far more pain in the future.

**Possible side effects:** None known, but there is also no scientific evidence that CMO is safe to use.

## Collagen

As we mentioned in the section on glucosamine and chondroitin, collagen is a common substance found in humans and animals. A protein, it is the chief component of cartilage, that cushioning, rubbery substance essential to healthy joint movement. Collagen is also sold as collagen hydrolysate or gelatin. There are many gelatin supplements on the market. Collagen supplements are made from cartilage of pigs, cows, oxen, chickens or sheep. It's available as a capsule, tablet or powder.

Collagen supplements supposedly relieve pain, inflammation and stiffness in people with various forms of arthritis. As collagen is a main component of cartilage, people take collagen to repair deteriorated cartilage also. But scientific evidence supporting these claims is controversial at this point. One recent study found that pharmaceutical-grade collagen hydrolysate did not relieve pain in people with bone or joint disease any better than a placebo. But studies are still ongoing.

**Possible side effects:** Stomach upset and nausea. People with allergies to chicken or eggs should not take collagen supplements made from chickens.

## Devil's Claw

Devil's claw, also known as grapple plant or wood spider, is made from a plant found in Namibia and South Africa. The supplement contains the active ingredient harpagoside, which appears to reduce pain and inflammation in some joints.

It's sold in capsule, powdered root or tea form. Devil's claw may not just relieve pain and inflammation, but also may serve as a digestive aid or appetite stimulant, something that may appeal to people with chronic pain or fatigue who may have lost their appetites. Some studies suggest that your stomach acid may counteract the beneficial ingredient, so it's advisable to take devil's claw between meals when stomach acid is at its lowest levels.

A recent clinical in vivo study on humans showed that devil's claw relieved hip and knee osteoarthritis pain, especially when used in conjunction with NSAIDs. The study also suggested that people using devil's claw may be able to decrease the amount of NSAIDs they take.

**Possible side effects:** Diarrhea. May affect heart rate and interfere with cardiac, blood-thinning or diabetes medicines. People with ulcers, gallstones or those taking antacids should not use devil's claw.

## Dimethyl Sulfoxide (DMSO)

DMSO is an organic liquid that is a byproduct of wood processing. It's used as an industrial solvent. In the early 1960s, DMSO gained a reputation as a new therapy for all forms of arthritis, and was believed to relieve pain and inflammation, and improve joint mobility. DMSO is available in cream, gel, injection, liquid or solution form. You should only take DMSO internally with a doctor's prescription. In the United States, DMSO is approved for treatment of the bladder condition interstitial cystitis, but does it relieve chronic pain and inflammation? Controlled studies of the topical forms of DMSO show mixed results.

**Possible side effects:** Headache, dizziness, drowsiness, nausea, vomiting, diarrhea, constipation and anorexia. Topical DMSO can cause skin irritations or dermatitis.

## Feverfew

Feverfew is made from the fresh or dried leaves of the feverfew plant commonly found in Europe. Available in capsule, tablet, fresh or dried leaf form, feverfew is supposed to relieve pain and inflammation.

Animal studies show that feverfew may reduce inflammation, but human studies show no benefit for people with arthritis.

**Possible side effects:** Stomach upset, diarrhea, flatulence and vomiting. In chewable form, feverfew may cause mouth sores, swelling of the mouth, tongue or lips, and loss of taste. People with allergies to plants in the daisy family (ragweed and marigolds) should avoid feverfew.

## Flaxseed

Flaxseed, flaxseed oil or linseed oil is a very common food additive made from the seed of the flax plant. (Flax is also the source of the fabric linen.) Flaxseed is available as whole seeds, oil, capsules or as ground meal or flour. You might add it to foods or take it with water. Flaxseed or flaxseed oil supposedly relieves joint pain and stiffness and lubricates joints for easier movement.

Flaxseed contains alpha-linolenic acid, an omega-3 fatty acid. This is a term you may hear frequently in the news. Omega-3 fatty acids are found in many food products, including some cold-water fish, like salmon or tuna. Omega-3 fatty acids have anti-inflammatory properties, one reason why doctors suggest adding these foods to your diet.

Flaxseed is also a natural laxative, so you should take this supplement in gradually increasing amounts and use some caution. Studies also show that flaxseed can lower total and LDL cholesterol levels in the blood, reduce risk of heart disease and cancer, and is a good source of fiber, which aids regularity of bowel movements. No studies clearly show that flaxseed can decrease inflammation, but because it contains omega-3 fatty acids, which scientists do believe to be anti-inflammatory, there is some that it may hold these properties.

**Possible side effects:** Can act as a laxative and impair absorption of some medications. Flaxseed acts as a blood thinner, so if you take blood-thinning medications, aspirin or NSAIDs, ask your doctor if you should use flaxseed.

## Ginger

Ginger is a common spice added to many foods and used as an ingredient in baked goods and other cooked foods. Ginger supplements come from the dried or fresh root of the ginger plant, and are available in powder, extract, tincture, spice and oil form. They're widely available, and ginger root is sold in most supermarkets.

People use ginger supplements to decrease joint pain and reduce inflammation, as well as a protection against stomach ulcers and nausea. People taking NSAIDs, as we learned in Chapter Four, can experience terrible stomach upset, so adding a ginger supplement or chewing candied ginger may offer some relief. Ginger does contain active ingredients that have analgesic and anti-inflammatory properties, and the root has long been used as an anti-nausea aid. One double-blind, clinical study of a highly purified ginger extract showed that the supplement reduced knee osteoarthritis pain.

**Possible side effects:** Heartburn, diarrhea and stomach discomfort. Ginger supplements may interfere with blood-pressure, blood-thinning, heart, diabetes or antacid medicines. People with gallstones should not use ginger supplements.

## GLA

GLA, or gamma-linoleic acid, is an omega-6 fatty acid (a natural anti-inflammatory agent) found in various plant oils: evening primrose, black currant and borage. It is sold in capsule or oil form. People use GLA to reduce joint pain, swelling and stiffness, and to ease symptoms of some rheumatic diseases.

Studies show that GLA can reduce inflammation in people with rheumatoid arthritis with few side effects, and may help regulate the immune system. One placebo-controlled study of 56 people with active rheumatoid arthritis who used GLA for six months showed the participants experienced significant joint pain reduction and improvements in stiffness and grip strength.

**Possible side effects:** Evening primrose oil: Indigestion, nausea, soft stools and headache. Borage seed oil: May exacerbate liver disease. Any type of GLA should be used orally. GLA is a blood thinner, so people using NSAIDs, anticoagulant medication or other blood-thinning supplements may see increased risk of bleeding.

## Gotu Kola

Gotu kola, also known as gotu cola, brahmi, brahma-buti or Indian pennywort, comes from a plant, *centella asiatica,* that grows in India, Japan, China, South Africa and Indonesia. Gotu kola is available as a capsule, tablet, tincture, cream, ointment, dried leaf or tea. People take gotu kola to reduce pain and fatigue, and to improve circulation.

Gotu kola does contain ingredients that may have analgesic or anti-inflammatory effects, but there is little scientific evidence to support this claim. Early in vivo studies using animals suggest it may prevent or treat gastrointestinal ulcers, and as a topical cream, may help psoriasis. No clinical studies on humans support any of these claims.

**Possible side effects:** Stomach upset, nausea, drowsiness, sensitivity to sunlight, and increased blood pressure, glucose and cholesterol levels. Could interfere with high blood pressure or diabetes medications.

## Green Tea

Much has been written about the health benefits of green tea, a widely consumed beverage throughout Asia and increasingly, in the West. Green tea contains a substance that supposedly fights inflammation, and a concentrated version of this substance is available in capsule and tablet form. You also can buy and drink green tea in standard tea bags or loose leaves.

In some studies on animals, green tea has been shown to have anti-inflammatory benefits, and laboratory studies also showed some promise that green tea reduces inflammation and slows the breakdown of cartilage. Both inflammation and cartilage breakdown are common in arthritis and can lead to terrible pain. But no human studies have shown any confirmed benefit for taking green tea if you have arthritis.

**Possible side effects:** Stomach upset, constipation. Green tea contains caffeine, so take this fact into account if you are sensitive to caffeine, pregnant or nursing.

## MSM

MSM is another supplement receiving wide attention from the media in recent years for its purported pain-relieving effects. MSM (short for methylsulfonylmethane) is an organic sulfur compound found in many plants, animals and even in humans. This compound is necessary for the formation of connective tissue. In supplement form, it's available as a tablet, powder and topical ointment.

MSM supplements supposedly ease pain and inflammation. A few studies performed on animals support the notion that it eases inflammation, and early studies on humans show it may relieve symptoms of arthritis. But

more scientific, controlled studies are needed to be sure if MSM really works.

**Possible side effects:** None known at this time.

## New Zealand Green-Lipped Mussel

While you may dine on New Zealand green-lipped mussels at a fine restaurant, you may not know that a concentrated, freeze-dried, supplement version of the tasty shellfish is available as an alternative pain treatment. The mussels contain those inflammation-fighting omega-3 fatty acids as well as other substances, lyprinol and glycomarine, believed to lessen painful inflammation.

Studies suggest that glycomarine may be the key ingredient. Some studies have shown that people with osteoarthritis who take glycomarine see reduced inflammation and pain, and increased joint lubrication. But many product labels don't indicate if the brand of mussel supplement contains glycomarine. You might try contacting the manufacturer to see if their product contains glycomarine.

**Possible side effects:** Diarrhea, nausea, intestinal gas and liver problems. If you're allergic to shellfish, do not use.

## SAM-e

Like many supplements, SAM-e, short for S-adnosyl-L-methionine, occurs in nature. You can buy SAM-e in tablet form, but your doctor might also inject it. SAM-e has many purported benefits, including relief of pain, stiffness and joint swelling, improvement of joint mobility and easing depression. Many people with chronic pain conditions such as osteoarthritis, bursitis, tendinitis, fibromyalgia or lower back pain use SAM-e and consider it effective. In Europe, SAM-e is sold as a drug and most studies on the compound have been conducted there.

Studies suggest that SAM-e is effective at improving joint health and treating the painful symptoms of osteoarthritis. Other studies done in the laboratory and on animals suggest SAM-e might repair and rebuild damaged cartilage. SAM-e can be expensive, and it may take longer to relieve pain than NSAIDs.

**Possible side effects:** Flatulence, vomiting, diarrhea, headache and nausea, but mostly these effects are seen when one has taken high doses of SAM-e. Should be avoided by people with bipolar disorder or Parkinson's disease. Could interact with antidepressants.

## Sea Algae

One small study conducted recently suggested some pain-relief promise for an herbal supplement made from an extract of sea algae, a plant found naturally in ocean waters. Researchers process the algae and create an extract containing astaxanthin, which is an antioxidant.

Antioxidants are found in many foods and can help flush out destructive byproducts in the body. But scientists still don't know how to best harness antioxidants or how much antioxidant-rich food or supplements to ingest to receive benefits. Some believe a healthy diet of foods rich in antioxidants may be superior to taking pills or supplements.

Sea algae extract is supposed to relieve pain associated with arthritis and carpal tunnel syndrome, the increasingly common disorder that causes wrist and hand pain and numbness. The extracts purportedly also provides sunburn protection and other claims. Still, many more studies are needed to determine if sea algae extract works to help relieve pain.

**Possible side effects:** Shown to be safe when taken as directed.

## Shark Cartilage

Cartilage is the flexible but firm substance that cushions many joints and helps us move more freely. Sharks have mostly cartilage, one reason why the deep-sea predators move through the water with such ease and grace. Along with eating their meat and fins for dinner, people are using the fearsome fishes' cartilage as a nutritional supplement to ease pain and inflammation. It is ground and consumed as capsules, tablets, extract and powder.

Like other animals' cartilage, shark cartilage contains collagen, a substance known for its ability to reduce pain and inflammation. It also contains calcium, a mineral known for its bone-building properties. Shark cartilage also contains chondroitin sulfate, which is used as a pain-and-inflammation-fighting supplement on its own (see p. 118). Some people with psoriasis, a painful condition affecting the skin and sometimes, joints and internal organs, use shark cartilage in an ointment form, applied on skin rashes. Some early studies on animals and in laboratories suggest shark cartilage may be effective in reducing pain and inflammation.

**Possible side effects:** Dizziness, nausea, vomiting, stomach upset, constipation, stomach bloating, fatigue, low blood pressure, high blood sugar and high calcium levels.

## Stinging Nettle

This supplement used for pain relief sounds painful itself. In fact, if you touch the leaves of a stinging nettle plant, you'll feel a "sting" and a skin irritation. Tiny, hairlike fibers on the leaves contain chemicals that bother the skin, but may also relieve pain in a counterirritant fashion.

This common treatment is made from the stinging nettle plant's leaves and roots, and you consume it as a tea, tincture or extract, or use the leaves to apply directly to your skin. People with osteoarthritis use stinging nettle to relieve pain, aches and inflammation. Some studies suggest that stinging nettle supplements may be taken in conjunction with NSAIDs to relieve pain, possibly allowing some to reduce their NSAID dose.

**Possible side effects:** Can increase blood clotting and effects of tranquilizers or sedatives, and can decrease effectiveness of blood thinners, diabetes or heart medications.

## Thunder God Vine

This dramatic-sounding supplement is an extract made from the leaf and root of an Asian plant. Thunder god vine (scientific name *tripterygium wilfordii Hook F*) extract supposedly relieves pain, inflammation and other symptoms in people with serious autoimmune disorders like rheumatoid arthritis and lupus.

Few studies have been performed on humans to determine the effectiveness of thunder god vine. A recent small study by doctors at the NIH reported that their subjects, who had rheumatoid arthritis, experienced a reduction in symptoms compared to those who took a placebo supplement. One Chinese study on people with rheumatoid arthritis also taking NSAIDs found that the extract helped relieve symptoms. Another Chinese study showed promise for the supplement in treating lupus symptoms.

Yet this supplement may be dangerous for many people whom it's supposed to help. People taking immune system suppressing drugs like prednisone (a drug many people with inflammatory forms of arthritis or other autoimmune diseases take) should not use extract of thunder god vine, as it could further suppress their immune systems. The leaves and flowers of the thunder god vine are poisonous, so only use extracts made from the plant's roots.

**Possible side effects:** Stomach upset, hair loss, heartburn, diarrhea, skin reactions, loss of menstruation in women and temporary infertility in men.

## Turmeric

Like ginger, turmeric is a commonly used spice added to many foods, such as curry. Made from a plant grown in India and Indonesia, it's a common ingredient in cuisines of those countries. Turmeric is related to the ginger family of plants. As a supplement, you may take it in capsule or powder form.

Turmeric is used to reduce pain and inflam-

## KAVA: A POSSIBLY RISKY SUPPLEMENT

The FDA recently issued a statement about the risk of taking the popular nutritional supplement kava, also known as kava kava. Made from the dried root of the kava plant found in the Pacific islands and related to the pepper family, kava supposedly eased pain and depression. People drank kava as a brew or mixed it into a smoothie, or consumed it in capsule, tablet or powder form.

Kava affects the brain and central nervous system, where pain is felt. It also reduces stress and anxiety. But kava's side effects make it dangerous to use. Health authorities in many countries reported cases of liver problems linked to kava use, including cirrhosis, hepatitis and liver failure. While kava-linked liver damage seems rare at this point, the FDA still felt that the risk merited this announcement. For more information, log onto the FDA Web site at www.fda.gov or the National Center for Complementary and Alternative Medicine, http://nccam.nih.gov.

---

mation and to treat painful bursitis. It's a staple of Chinese and Indian Ayurvedic (traditional) medicine as an arthritis treatment and also as a digestive aid or body-cleansing agent. It may be used in combination with other common supplements. In fact, the only studies performed on turmeric have shown it may be effective in relieving arthritis-related pain when combined with boswellia, zinc, ginger or aswangandha (an Indian herbal treatment).

**Possible side effects:** Could cause stomach upset or thinning of blood when taken at high doses. If you have gallstones, do not use turmeric.

## Willow Bark

Aspirin was first created from the bark of the willow, a beautiful tree common to many parts of the world. The active ingredient in the supplemental form of willow bark (or white willow) is salicin, which is very similar to salicylates, the active chemical in aspirin. People with arthritis, gout, ankylosing spondylitis, back problems and other painful arthritis-related diseases use willow bark to ease muscle and joint aches and pains.

The drawback may be that it takes a great deal of willow bark to get enough of the pain-fighting ingredient, so it may be easier to take an aspirin. You might have to take willow bark tea or extract much longer to get the same benefit as aspirin pills. Willow bark is also available in a cream form for treating minor skin irritations. But one study did show that it provided pain relief for people with osteoarthritis and low back pain.

**Possible side effects:** Similar to aspirin. Can increase the effect of blood thinners. Should not be used by children under 18 due to risk of Reye's syndrome.

## SUPPLEMENTS FOR FIBROMYALGIA

People with fibromyalgia often experience a combination of symptoms, including muscle pain, aches, fatigue, sleeplessness and depression or anxiety. Because the root cause of fibromyalgia is not known at this time, the disease can be hard to treat. Doctors usually respond by prescribing drugs to treat fibromyalgia's various symptoms. Supplements used by people with fibromyalgia often address sleep problems and mood-related symptoms.

If you have fibromyalgia, you may be curious about exploring natural supplements that may ease these symptoms as well. Here are several popular supplements for fibromyalgia symptoms. As we noted earlier in this chapter, inform your doctor if you wish to try one of these supplements. Some supplements may compound the effects of your prescribed drugs and cause problems. Note: SAM-e, described on p. 124, is also used by people with fibromyalgia to ease depression.

### Ginseng

Many people throughout Asia use ginseng, a plant root, for various health benefits, including relief from stress and fatigue, a boost to the immune system, increase in physical stamina and cognitive function – all benefits that might appeal to a person with fibromyalgia. Reports say that as many as six million Americans use ginseng regularly for various health reasons.

Sold as a fresh root or ground up in capsule, tablet, tea, tincture powder or tonic form, scientists do not know how or if ginseng really works. Few studies have been done and those that have show little true benefit.

**Possible side effects:** Ginseng can increase the effects of corticosteroid medicines like prednisone. It can also cause insomnia, something people with fibromyalgia may be concerned about already, or act as a stimulant. People with heart conditions, hormone-sensitive conditions, diabetes, hypertension, low blood pressure or schizophrenia should avoid ginseng. Pregnant women, people who have had organ transplants, or people taking blood thinners, immunosuppressants or MAO inhibitors should avoid ginseng.

### Grapeseed

Grapeseed extract or oil supplements come from the seeds of Asian grapes, and people can take it in tablet or capsule form. Grapeseed oil supposedly fights inflammation, improves circulation, and also relieves symptoms of fibromyalgia and chronic fatigue syndrome, a similar condition marked by severe, ongoing weariness.

Grapeseed oil is a powerful antioxidant, and it contains vitamin E, flavonoids and essential fatty acids, all substances known to be important to overall health. But no studies prove its actual effectiveness for people with fibromyalgia.

**Possible side effects:** Can increase risk of bleeding, so do not use if you are using blood thinners or other supplements that have this action.

## Melatonin

Most people with fibromyalgia report trouble sleeping, and this lack of deep sleep may be one cause of their chronic pain. The body needs REM or deep sleep to rejuvenate its processes and restore energy for the coming day. People with fibromyalgia often don't get proper sleep, sparking a cycle of pain, fatigue and depression.

Melatonin is a widely popular herbal sleep aid sold in nearly every drugstore and supermarket. The supplement is derived from an animal version of a hormone found also in humans' pineal glands, located at the base of the brain. It comes in capsule, tablet, liquid, lozenge or tea form.

Melatonin is a powerful antioxidant, and it regulates the human sleep cycle to treat insomnia or restless, disturbed sleep common in fibromyalgia. Taking aspirin and other NSAIDs may lower natural melatonin levels. Studies suggest that melatonin may boost the immune system and bone growth, but no valid clinical studies prove its effectiveness as a sleep aid. However, it is widely used as a sleep aid. Doctors suggest that people should use melatonin as a short-term aid.

**Possible side effects:** May interact with heart or depression medicines and immuno-suppressants. Don't mix with alcohol as it could dangerously intensify the effect, and do not take along with similar sleep-promoting supplements such as valerian.

## St. John's Wort

This popular mood-boosting supplement is an extract of a wild plant with yellow flowers, St. John's wort, which grows in the U.S. and Europe. It's sold in powder, liquid, tablet, capsule or tea form.

People take St. John's wort as an antidepressant and to reduce muscle pain common in fibromyalgia. Researchers believe the plant contains active ingredients that boost levels of serotonin, a brain chemical that may be linked to the pain, sensitivity and sleep problems of fibromyalgia. People need to take St. John's wort for up to a month to see its benefits, and they may experience withdrawal symptoms if they suddenly stop taking the supplement.

St. John's wort may relieve mild to moderate, but not severe, depression. You should only take St. John's wort with your doctor's approval as it can interact with some medications. St. John's wort should not be taken by people taking antidepressants. In such cases, the supplement could compound the effects of the drugs.

**Possible side effects:** Sensitivity to sunlight, dizziness, insomnia, fatigue, anxiety, stomach upset and dry mouth.

## Valerian Root

A popular herbal sleep aid, valerian root or valerian is used widely in Europe and increasingly in the United States to ease sleeplessness and to ease muscle and joint pain. Valerian, a pungent, ground plant root, is sold in capsule, tablet, extract or tea form. Valerian teas are very strong-tasting and may be unpalatable to some people.

Valerian is a mild sedative and aids sleep without the grogginess of many prescription sedatives. Clinical studies suggest it is an effective insomnia treatment, but no studies prove its effectiveness for pain relief. Do not take with alcohol or other sedatives as it might intensify the effects.

**Possible side effects:** In some cases, valerian does not work at all to relieve insomnia and has the opposite effect, causing sleeplessness, headache, excitability or an uneasy feeling.

## VITAMINS, MINERALS AND DIETARY CHANGES

Many doctors and health-care professionals suggest a diet rich in vitamins, minerals and nutrients for good health. Can a higher intake of certain vitamins and minerals – or even a change in what foods you eat – cause or lessen your pain? It's not likely that popping a particular vitamin pill each day will truly relieve pain, but research does show the power of certain nutrients to control painful diseases like arthritis, osteoporosis and more.

In addition, some people subscribe to a theory that particular diets will help control pain and inflammation. There is not enough evidence to support these theories, but there are safe, healthy ways to test if certain foods trigger or worsen your pain.

One chronic pain condition clearly linked to the content of your diet is gout. People with gout should follow a specific diet that eliminates or greatly reduces consumption of foods high in purines. For most people, doctors and health experts recommend a varied diet, rich in vitamins, minerals and nutrients, and low in fatty or processed foods. If you do have a chronic pain condition, you may wish to make an effort to include foods rich in particular nutrients, such as omega-3 fatty acids (common in cold-water fish) that can fight inflammation, or foods rich in antioxidants, nutrients that help fight the effects of *free radicals,* molecules in the environment that play a role in the aging and disease processes.

### Gout and Diet

Gout, which usually results from a high uric acid level in the blood, is one of the few chronic pain conditions that clearly can be helped by cutting back on certain foods. However, since drugs like allopurinol and probenecid work so well to control painful gout attacks, some people with gout may rely on their drugs to control the pain rather than avoiding what may have caused the pain in the first place: their purine-rich diets.

People with gout can lower uric acid levels in their blood through several steps. One, they can avoid foods high in purines, including meats, poultry, organ meats like liver or kidneys, dried beans or peas, herring, mackerel, scallops, sardines, anchovies, and even vegetables like asparagus, spinach, cauliflower and mushrooms.

There are a few other steps to reduce the chances of a gout attack:

- **Don't drink alcoholic beverages**, as they may increase uric acid levels in the blood.
- **Don't fast**, as this action could increase uric acid levels in the blood and trigger an attack.
- **Control your weight**, but reduce excess weight gradually.
- **Drink plenty of water** – as much as two to three quarts daily – so your kidneys can flush properly and excrete uric acid.

## Is Food a Pain Trigger?

Could certain foods be pain triggers or disease fighters? Experts have not yet confirmed this to be true, but more information is being discovered about the links between nutrition and disease.

One chronic pain condition triggered by certain foods is headaches, such as migraine headaches. People with chronic headaches should consider avoiding trigger foods, including chocolate, red wine or red wine vinegars, the seasoning monosodium glutamate, aged cheeses, processed meats, and foods or beverages containing caffeine.

Scientists believe that a small percentage of the population suffers from true food allergies, where even a small amount of a certain food elicits a serious physical reaction. But many people may be sensitive to certain foods. If they have a chronic pain condition, eating certain foods could make them feel worse. If a person has a chronic inflammatory condition, a diet high in foods like saturated animal fats and many vegetable oils might contribute to joint and tissue inflammation that causes serious pain.

In the past, many "arthritis diets" have circulated, perpetuated further by the creation of the Internet. These diets claim to cure arthritis or greatly reduce pain simply by eliminating certain foods. These claims are unproven. Unlike the headache triggers, no particular food has been proven to trigger joint pain, arthritis or inflammation.

However, two facts about diet and arthritis are true. One, if you are overweight, you increase your risk of developing osteoarthritis or making any type of arthritis worse. Excess weight puts additional strain on joints, and if your joints are damaged or weakened due to arthritis, they don't need excess strain. Two, there are some reports that support the idea that certain nutrients (including particular oils, vegetables and animal products) may either help or worsen joint pain. Some doctors might suggest you use more "good" oils such as olive, canola or flaxseed, and less "bad" oils, such as corn or safflower, in your diet. Oils rich in omega-6 fatty acids may contribute to inflammation, while oils rich in omega-3 linoleic fatty acids (found in cold-water fish, flaxseed oil and other foods) may be beneficial to people with inflammation.

Many Internet sites and magazine stories promote the idea of adopting extreme diets as a way to fight disease. Switching from your balanced diet to a radically different diet lacking whole food groups may do more harm than good, depriving you of important nutrients. Some diets promote certain combinations of foods as magic "cures" for arthritis or chronic pain, but there is no evidence to support such claims.

At this time, theories linking foods to pain or inflammation are just that: theories. Only hearsay and uncontrolled studies provide any basis for these theories. Since many people with chronic pain have serious or systemic illnesses, it's difficult to determine what may cause their flares. Certain foods, such as spicy, greasy, high-fiber or hard-to-digest foods, may cause stomach upset or gas. This can be painful and can disrupt sleep. Poor sleep can worsen pain for many people.

Some research does support the link between food and pain. Red meat and many vegetable oils, including corn, sunflower and safflower oils, break down into arachidonic acids in the body. These acids are building blocks for prostaglandins and leukotrienes that can cause pain and inflammation. It is possible to eat a diet free of some of these foods by choosing poultry, fish or vegetarian meals and using olive or canola oils for cooking. You might improve your heart's health and your weight in the process. Another theory is the "leaky gut" syndrome. This theory contends that some diseases, including arthritis, fibromyalgia, Crohn's disease and others, may cause the intestines to become leaky or porous, allowing tiny molecules from foods or bacteria to slip through to the rest of the body. The theory is that the leaks lead to inflammation, pain and exacerbated immune system problems. Studies have not yet confirmed if leaky gut syndrome is real.

How can you tell if a certain food may be causing or worsening your pain? Keep a food diary. Take note of everything you eat for at least one week. Make sure you note the various ingredients of your foods. Read labels of different products you use and ask questions about the foods you eat in restaurants. Take note of foods, seasonings or additives used in various dishes, including sauces. Write down what alcoholic beverages you consume and how much. Make sure you note the date and time when you ate or drank these items.

Also take note of when you experienced pain. Did a painful flare occur just after eating a particular meal? What did that meal contain? Watch for times when you ate other meals containing those ingredients. If you detect a pattern, try eliminating that one ingredient from your diet for a week or two. See if your pain subsides. On the flip side, you might try adding certain foods, like the oils listed earlier (see p. 131), in moderate amounts and keeping track of any beneficial changes you detect over time.

What foods are the most commonly reported triggers of pain? This is not true for every person experiencing pain or inflammation, but here is a short list:

Dairy foods. Some people may be *lactose intolerant,* or lacking the enzyme to break down lactase in dairy foods like milk, cheese, butter or cream. These people may experience painful gas, cramps or diarrhea after eating these foods. Some people believe that dairy foods can worsen inflammatory forms of arthritis. While this is not proven, you can try a dairy-free diet without sacrificing nutrition. It is important to maintain healthy levels of calcium with soy, vegetables and other foods, or calcium supplements.

Nightshade vegetables. Some people believe that eating vegetables in the *Solanaceae* or nightshade family lead to joint inflammation. These foods include tomatoes, potatoes, eggplant and peppers. Horticulturist Norman F. Childers, Ph.D., first proposed this theory; his diverticulitis (a painful inflammation of part of the intestines) and flared after he ate nightshade vegetables. He conducted one seven-year, uncontrolled, large study of people with arthritis who avoided eating these vegetables; the study found that nearly 75 percent of the people saw decreased pain and disability. However, many doctors believe the nightshade theory is speculative at best and may be completely untrue.

Food additives or seasonings. Additives or seasonings like monosodium glutamate (MSG), nitrates or salt may cause unpleasant or painful reactions in some people. These additives are common in processed or packaged foods, cured meats like bacon or luncheon meat, and meals prepared in restaurants.

Other purported pain triggers. Red meat, pork, eggs, peanuts, coffee, wheat, aspartame and corn have all been mentioned as possible triggers of pain. Scientific evidence has not proven that these foods do lead to flares of pain. If you believe eating these foods has contributed to flares of your pain, talk to your doctor before eliminating anything from your diet or assuming you have an "allergy" to these foods.

Diets that eliminate whole groups of foods – such as all carbohydrates, vegetables, fruits, fats or proteins – are not considered healthy eating plans by most nutritionists. It's important to eat a diet that is balanced, so you receive all the nutrients your body needs to run properly. For example, if you choose a vegetarian diet in an effort to lose weight or improve your health, you need to compensate for the eliminated meat protein with plant-based proteins, such as tofu or beans.

Another common pain-fighting practice that could be dangerous to your health is fasting, or abstaining from food for a period of time. Some fasts allow the person to only drink water or fruit juice for several days. The theory behind fasting as a therapy is that the fast cleanses the body of toxins or any foods that may have caused pain. After the fast, the person then starts adding one food at a time until they determine what foods may cause pain.

It is not recommended to fast for any period of time if you have a chronic illness or chronic pain. This is especially true if you are taking medications for pain. Don't fast unless your doctor specifically advises you to abstain from food (such as if you are having surgery or undergoing a certain test). Fasting could only lead to weakness, dizziness, dehydration and other problems. Fasting can trigger attacks in people with gout.

What about foods you might add to your diet to increase joint health or decrease pain? Could certain vitamin or nutrient supplements help as well? Striking the right balance of oils and omega fatty acids in your diet may help fight inflammation. Canola and olive oils also have a better balance of good fatty acids than corn, sunflower or safflower oil, which are high in omega-6 fatty acids and can lead to inflammation. Using small amounts of canola and olive oil in your food preparation can also encourage better heart health.

Some people take fish oil supplements instead of eating a lot of fish meals to get the health benefits of the omega-3 fatty acids. They can also add flaxseed to their foods. Flaxseed can act as a laxative; use it with this in mind. Gamma-linolenic acid (GLA), usually taken in supplement form as borage oil, evening primrose oil or black currant seed oil, can also help fight painful inflammation. GLA can aid in the body's production of series 1-prostaglandins, which can fight inflammation.

## Vitamins and Minerals

The idea of "taking your vitamins" suggests that getting the right nutrients, whether through a balanced diet or a supplement, can boost good health. Some people believe that doses of certain vitamins can prevent or treat illness as well. Research is beginning to prove them right in certain cases, although using vitamins in the same way we use drugs is not likely to offer pain relief.

What is a vitamin? Vitamins are natural substances present in plant and animal foods. The word "vitamin" was first used by Polish biochemist Casimir Funk in the early 20th century. Dr. Funk studied chickens that developed a nerve inflammation or neuritis. Dr. Funk discovered that the cause of the inflammation was a lack of a certain nutrient in the chickens' diet. Dr. Funk named the nutrient a "vitamine," combining the Latin term *vita*, or life, with the word *amine*, referring to chemical compounds that contain nitrogen (we now know vitamins don't have to contain nitrogen). Later, newly discovered vitamins were identified with letters of the alphabet: A, B, C, D, E, K and so on.

Minerals are inorganic substances that come from the earth. Many minerals, such as iron, selenium, zinc and calcium, are necessary for the body's growth and the normal functioning of many body processes. When we have a severe lack of important minerals, physical sickness can result. Many multivitamin supplements contain a mixture of vitamins and minerals that are designed to make up for any deficiencies in your dietary intake of these nutrients. However, it is always preferable to get your vitamins and minerals from a healthy, varied diet rather than from a pill. Your doctor may determine that you need additional supplements of certain vitamins or minerals for disease prevention or good health.

Can vitamin or mineral supplements ease pain? It's unlikely, but with a doctor's supervision, these supplements can be part of an overall disease-prevention and pain-management plan. Some vitamins and minerals help prevent *cell oxidation*. Oxidation is a natural process that means any substance is combining with oxygen, present throughout the atmosphere. When metal rusts, the substance of the metal is combining with the air around it, and the oxidation results in rust. While the process of cells oxidizing isn't the same as your body rusting from within, it is true that cells can break down in the oxidation process. Certain vitamins and other nutrients work as antioxidants. Antioxidants can help prevent the cell breakdown that could lead to serious, painful diseases like arthritis or cancer.

While you can take multivitamin supplements or vitamin and mineral pills that contain antioxidants, it's best to get most of your nutrients from the foods you eat. When you eat a varied diet of fresh foods, you are more likely to get all the vitamins you need, along with fiber, iron and other important nutrients. Multivitamin supplements can complement a healthy diet, but shouldn't replace it. Antioxidants and good food sources of these nutrients include:

- **Beta-carotene:** Carrots, sweet potatoes and leafy, green vegetables
- **Vitamin C:** Citrus fruits, berries, tomatoes, and most vegetables
- **Vitamin E:** Nuts, leafy, green vegetables, wheat germ, liver and sweet potatoes
- **Selenium:** Seafood, organ meats, and some grains and seeds

Vitamin D is another important nutrient that may help people with chronic pain conditions, including osteoarthritis. Vitamin D is commonly found in dairy products enriched with the vitamin. Low levels of vitamin D have been found in people with osteoarthritis, so these people may need to supplement the nutrient. In addition, when you are outside during the day and exposed to sunlight, your body synthesizes vitamin D. People with

chronic pain may not get outdoors regularly, especially if their pain keeps them in bed or on the couch. They may get even less sunlight exposure during cold, winter months when the weather may be bad and there are fewer hours of daylight. This lack of sun exposure can lead to more fatigue, as there are proven links between vitamin D and healthy sleep and energy levels. Supplements of the vitamin and new, safe sunlight lamps may be helpful.

Is illness caused by a lack of vitamins or minerals? Diseases like scurvy and beriberi once plagued people who had a complete lack of certain vitamins in their diet, but today, such diseases caused by vitamin deficiency are very rare. However, a lack of essential vitamins and minerals in your diet could be a contributing factor to the development of more common diseases like arthritis, osteoporosis, heart disease and cancer.

We've already discussed important antioxidants to include in your diet. There are other nutrients that are essential to eat enough of: calcium and iron. Calcium helps you build strong bones. Good sources of calcium include milk or dairy products, fortified cereals or juices, leafy green vegetables and canned sardines or salmon with bones. Iron is also essential to good health and the prevention of anemia, a lower than normal count of red blood cells. People with anemia can experience fatigue and tire easily.

Over the years, more research has been conducted about these possible links between a lack of certain vitamins and various health problems. For example, a person who does not get enough calcium in their diet is at a higher risk for developing osteoporosis. People with osteoarthritis often show lower levels of vitamins C and D in their bodies.

The question that follows is: Can taking extra amounts of certain vitamins prevent or relieve painful conditions? Most doctors don't recommend taking high doses of particular vitamins, at least not without a doctor's supervision. Overuse of vitamin or mineral supplements, even ones you may consider healthful, could lead to other health problems. Overdose of some vitamins is possible and could be toxic. So it's important to only take vitamins or minerals after clearing it with your doctor.

If you take aspirin or other NSAIDs for your pain, don't take your medicine at the same time you take your vitamin. Aspirin and other NSAIDs can cause vitamins and other supplements to break down more quickly and easily, decreasing their effectiveness. Take your vitamin or other supplements 2-3 hours before or after you take your NSAID.

It's also important for people with any chronic illness or chronic pain condition to have a nutritious diet and take vitamin supplements if necessary. Some medications used by people with chronic illness (who may take these drugs over a long period of time) may lower the amount of certain nutrients in your body. For example, methotrexate, a drug taken by many people with rheumatoid arthritis, severe asthma, cancer and other diseases, may lower levels of folic acid, an important nutrient, in the body. Folic acid (found in many enriched breakfast cereals) helps prevent birth defects, but it also plays a key role in the production of SAM (see p. 124) in the body, which helps maintain healthy cartilage. Folic acid supplements may lower the severity or frequency of the serious side effects of methotrexate, so there is an added benefit to taking this supplement while on methotrexate.

Many people with chronic illness show a lack of certain nutrients in their blood, and they may not get enough exercise or eat a proper diet due to fatigue, depression, side effects of medications or constant pain. So nutritional supplements may be helpful in boosting overall wellness, energy and perhaps ease pain or other symptoms.

The link between vitamins and minerals and disease is complex. It's important not to try to treat yourself with nutritional supplements, but instead to rely on the advice of your doctor. Ask your doctor if you should merely take a multivitamin supplement or if you need concentrated amounts of a particular vitamin or mineral. Chances are good that the best approach will be a broad one, with a healthy diet, regular exercise and proper medications.

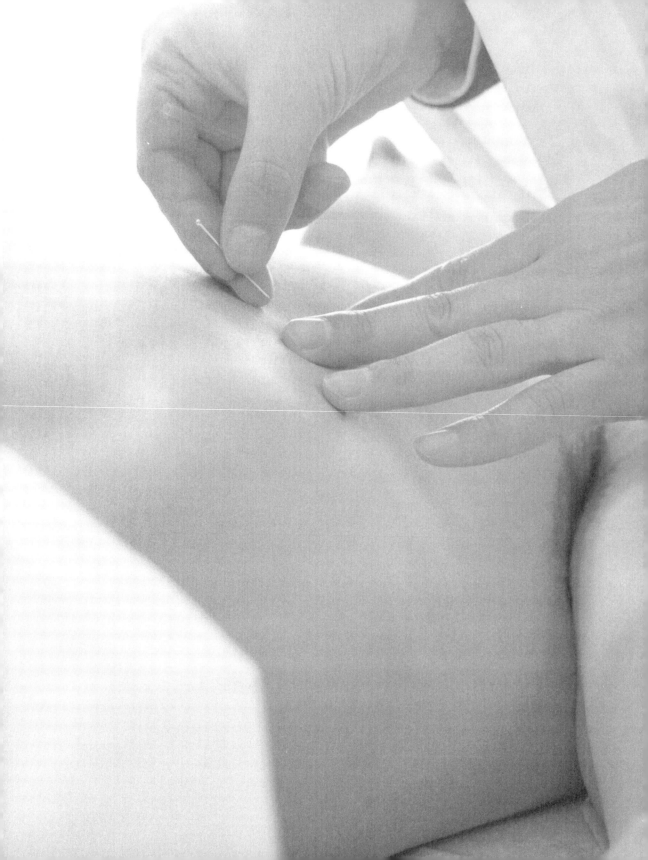

# Massage, Manipulation and Other Alternatives

8

# CHAPTER 8: MASSAGE, MANIPULATION AND OTHER ALTERNATIVES

Some alternative therapies for pain relief don't involve taking herbs or nutritional supplements. There are many alternative philosophies of healing, as well as treatments performed by practitioners of these philosophies, that are increasing in popularity for people with chronic pain.

Some of these treatments rise from ancient healing traditions in China or India. Others stem from relatively recent health philosophies developed in the United States. No matter how old or new these alternative treatments are, they tend to spark controversy, as well as debate among doctors and their patients.

No matter what therapy you try, it's important to find out if the practitioner is licensed by state or national boards and has the proper training to perform the procedures. Never allow a practitioner who is not properly licensed to perform any type of manipulation or treatment on your body. You should also consult your insurance policy before any appointment with a chiropractor, acupuncturist, massage therapist or alternative therapy practitioner to see if the treatment is covered. If it is not, agree on fees and terms beforehand so you will know what charges you will owe for these services.

Consult your primary-care doctor also so he knows what therapies you are exploring. In some cases, your doctor can refer you to reputable, qualified practitioners of various therapies. Some doctors also perform the following therapies as part of their integrative practice. In addition, some physical therapists, occupational therapists or other health-care professionals may offer some of these services.

## ACUPUNCTURE AND ACUPRESSURE

Acupuncture is an ancient, Asian healing technique that has gained popularity in the West over the past few decades. A 1998 Harvard University study showed that Americans may make as many as five million visits to acupuncturists yearly. Mainstream medical institutions now take acupuncture seriously and are studying the therapy to determine why and how well it works. The National Institutes of Health (NIH) has funded research on acupuncture to explore its effectiveness.

Acupuncture is part of a type of alternative medicine called *Chinese medicine.* Chinese medicine, which may also involve herbs, massage, meditation techniques or exercises, developed over thousands of years in China, but has gained new popularity in the United States in recent years. One of the main reasons people in the West seek acupuncture treatment is to relieve chronic pain, especially back pain, arthritis or fibromyalgia. The FDA approved special acupuncture needles for use by licensed acupuncture practitioners in 1996, so there is some regulation of the equipment used in this procedure. Currently, a number of legitimate, scientific studies are being conducted to research the effectiveness and safety of acupuncture treatment specifically for osteoarthritis and other diseases involving chronic pain.

Acupuncture involves a trained professional puncturing the skin with very thin needles at any of 300 specific sites on the body. These points lay along energy pathways call *meridians.* Devotees of acupuncture believe that puncturing (very lightly; you should not feel pain from the puncture) the body at these points will increase the energy flow (called qi; pronounced *chee*) along the meridians. Qi is, in traditional Chinese belief, essential to healthy balance in the body, known as yin and yang.

Acupuncture supposedly boosts the body's natural ability to heal itself and relieve pain. *Acupressure* is another form of this treatment, but one involving hand pressure rather than needle punctures. Acupuncturists follow an ancient, specific map of the body that shows particular places to prick to relieve pain in other areas.

Studies about acupuncture show some merit to these claims. They find that some people have higher production of endorphins, those natural pain-fighting chemicals the body produces, in their cerebrospinal fluid after acupuncture.

Scientists do not yet understand why pricking the skin at these particular points causes the endorphin boost, or why acupuncturists stick the flesh at a particular point to stimulate pain relief in a completely different part of the body. Acupuncture may stimulate the flow of electromagnetic signals through the body along the meridians, helping endorphins flow. Acupuncture may also activate the release of the central nervous system's natural opioids (similar to the chemicals in narcotic drugs), which relieve pain and boost sleep. Or it may aid in the release of certain neurotransmitters, body chemicals that play a role in how the brain relays pain messages, and *neurohormones*, more brain chemicals that can affect the structure or function of the body's organs.

More scientific studies are necessary if acupuncture is to be established as a confirmed pain-relief treatment, but the NIH has issued statements about the promising results of various studies and the procedure's possible efficacy in treating many painful conditions, including headache, tennis elbow, fibromyalgia, myofascial pain, osteoarthritis, low back pain, carpal tunnel syndrome and more. Most doctors who support the use of acupuncture believe it should be used as a complement to regular medical treatment of chronic pain. Many states have licensing boards that license acupuncturists and other individuals who practice "healing arts" to perform treatments. Contact your secretary of state's office to see if your state has such a board.

What Happens During Acupuncture? During an acupuncture session, the practitioner (known as an acupuncturist) will insert the needles and leave them resting in the body while you lie on a table for about 20 minutes. (In acupressure, he applies pressure to these points.) He may move them to other points on the body depending on your painful problem. Then he will likely remove the needles and ask you to rest some more before rising from the table. Reactions to the procedure vary widely from person to person. Usually, repeated treatments are needed for relief of chronic pain.

Some acupuncturists also use electrical stimulation in the needles to boost the procedure's effects, a procedure known as *electroacupuncture*. Others use dried herbs (in the U.S., compressed sticks of these herbs) as part of their treatment of the patient, a practice called *moxibustion*.

To find an acupuncturist in your area, first ask your doctor for a referral. If he cannot give you any information, consult the National Certification Commission for Acupuncture and Oriental Medicine, the national body that certifies acupuncturists. They can be reached at (703) 548-9004 or online at www.nccaom.org.

## MANIPULATION THERAPIES

One popular treatment for pain relief, particularly of chronic neck and back pain or post-injury pain, is *manipulation therapy,* or manual adjustment of the spine or the limbs in order to restore proper alignment or promote the body's natural healing ability. Many different health-care professionals perform manipulation therapy, and the therapy they offer may vary slightly from discipline to discipline. Chiropractors are probably the most common practitioners of this therapy, but osteopaths, physical therapists and even some medical doctors may also perform it.

## Chiropractic

Millions of Americans each year visit *doctors of chiropractic* for pain treatment and other health-care needs. Chiropractic is a belief system that holds that pain and many other health problems, including minor and serious diseases, occur because the body's spine is out of alignment, a condition they call *vertebral subluxation.* Chiropractors, as these professionals are commonly called, perform regular adjustments to the spine, or *spinal manipulations,* in order to restore the spine to its optimal position. According to the philosophy of chiropractic, a well-adjusted spine allows the body to perform its natural defenses of pain and disease at optimal levels.

While there is dispute among scientists as to the validity of the theory of chiropractic, many people seek chiropractors and other health-care professionals for periodic or regular spinal manipulation as a therapy for pain. Whether or not the therapy works, or whether or not the philosophy behind it is valid, is a matter of opinion at this point.

Chiropractic began a little more than a century ago in Iowa, when a lay healer named David Daniel Palmer formed the basic theory of vertebral subluxations. His treatment philosophy spread. Today numerous chiropractic colleges train and license doctors of chiropractic to treat patients for pain and other ailments. The Council on Chiropractic Education is the organization that issues accreditation to chiropractic programs, and the American Chiropractic Association is the official professional organization of these practitioners. Chiropractors cannot prescribe drugs or perform surgery, but they do consult with patients and perform manipulation and other treatments.

Doctors of osteopathy, or osteopaths, are very similar to medical doctors. But osteopaths' philosophy of health and healing focuses often on the body's ability to heal itself than on doctor-administered drugs and other therapies.

Osteopathic medicine was founded in the 19th century, by a Civil War surgeon named Andrew Still, who was disillusioned by the failures of the mainstream medicine of his time. He devised his own theory that the body's musculoskeletal system was key to good health and the body's ability to defend itself against disease and heal itself following injury.

Osteopathy uses many of the same practices and follows many of the same principles as traditional or allopathic medicine. Osteopaths can prescribe drugs and perform surgery. Osteopathic medical schools put more emphasis on training their students for work as primary-care physicians or general practice, rather than medical specialties. In the examination room, osteopathic treatment may be quite similar to examinations by a medical doctor. However, osteopaths may focus more on general health and wellness practices, as well as addressing the home and work environment of the patient.

As osteopathic medicine is based on the idea that the musculoskeletal system is at the root of many diseases and pain conditions, osteopaths receive additional training in treating the mus-

culoskeletal system. Their treatment may include *osteopathic manipulative treatment,* using their hands on the body of the patient in an effort to diagnose disease, damage to tissues and more. Treatment by an osteopath may also include manipulation, where the doctor uses his hands more forcefully to correct problems in the musculoskeletal system.

### What Happens During Manipulation Therapy? 

Manipulation therapy usually follows a consultation with the practitioner and some diagnostic tests. Sometimes, the practitioner issues X-rays. Other tests may determine your range of motion (the amount of flexibility you have in certain joints), muscle tone or strength, reflexes and more. Then, the practitioner might perform the manipulation therapy, along with prescribing treatments and suggestions, such as herbal supplements, exercise or dietary changes.

Note: Be wary of any practitioner who issues excessive X-rays in order to diagnose your problem. This is unnecessary unless you have a serious bone disease, and could expose you to levels of radiation that are unhealthy. Do not be afraid to question your practitioner if he orders a series of X-rays without some valid explanation. You may have already had X-rays performed by your primary-care doctor, so offer to provide these images instead, or choose another practitioner. The practitioner should express willingness to address your concerns.

Spinal manipulation involves the practitioner using either his hands or a small pushing instrument to press on the spine, back and neck, or sometimes, the limbs. The manipulation often looks as if they are pushing or stretching your neck and back into alignment, while you lie on your stomach on a padded table. You may hear a crack or pop, but this is simply air being released from the moving vertebrae. The practitioner may have you rest for a few moments after the manipulation.

Study results and professional opinions are mixed on the benefit of spinal manipulation therapy for people with chronic pain. You may have to rely on your own judgment as to whether or not this therapy is worth trying. If you try spinal manipulation therapy and do not see some relief after three or four sessions, it probably won't work. You may receive some pain relief from the manipulations, but if you don't see improvement, try massage, water therapy, exercise or other techniques instead.

Be wary of any practitioner who claims that continual manipulations throughout your lifetime are necessary to achieving pain relief and good health; there is no evidence to support this claim. Also, be wary of any practitioner who suggests that you discontinue any other medical treatment or seeing your medical doctors for care.

Although it's likely that spinal manipulation is safe, people with inflammatory arthritis or osteoporosis should use caution as manipulation might damage weakened joints or bones. Fracture of bones can occur. It's essential to inform your chiropractor, osteopath, physical therapist or any other spinal manipulation practitioner about your health conditions. Don't just say, "I'm in pain." Practitioners need to know any possible health risks you may have in order to perform manipulation properly. If manipulation causes pain, stop the treatment and inform the practitioner.

## CranioSacral Therapy™

A similar form of manipulation therapy, although one less widely practiced, is *CranioSacral Therapy*™. This therapy aims to balance the fluids in what they term the craniosacral system, or the fluids that run down your spinal cord from the neck to the base of the spine. Practitioners and devotees believe an imbalance in this fluid can cause various health problems or pain.

In CranioSacral Therapy™, the practitioner stands behind you while you lie on a comfortable table, and gently holds your head in his hands while applying soft pressure to various points on the back of the neck. He may also apply gentle pressure to points at the base of the spine. Experts are very divided on the validity or usefulness of this procedure. Some people find it beneficial or relaxing.

Some chiropractors and osteopaths perform *cranial manipulation*, in which they apply gentle pressure to the skull in certain areas in order to relieve pain. They use the heels of their hands and press on particular points of the skull. Some professionals use this technique to relieve chronic neck and back pain, ear pain, and even *tinnitus*, or chronic ringing in the ears. Some of these practitioners believe that the cranial manipulation doesn't relieve the pain, but corrects misalignment of the skull's bones (which actually don't move) so the body's natural defense system can work more effectively.

## Somatic Therapy

Another chiropractic-related therapy for pain (and one that is really only performed by chiropractors) is *somatic therapy.* This therapy is based on a belief that muscles might weaken after an injury and not get back to normal because they "remember" the weakened position one might maintain in an effort to favor the painful body part (such as the back or a leg). Many chiropractors follow a theory called *kinesiology,* which focuses on the body's proper movement as a source of good health, and in somatic therapy, the practitioner performs a kinesiological examination to see if the person's muscles are performing incorrectly.

In somatic therapy, the practitioner guides the patient in a specific series of exercises that are meant to retrain the muscles, as well as the nerves and even the brain's response to the pain that may be guiding the muscles to behave incorrectly. The therapy, like many other chiropractic techniques, also involves some hands-on manipulation by the practitioner. The therapy aims to teach the muscles, nerves and the brain to act as they did before the injury, hopefully reducing pain. Somatic therapy is similar and inspired by the same beliefs as the *Alexander Technique* and *Feldenkrais Method,* two other common exercise-related or movement therapies that aim to reduce pain by "teaching" our bodies to move normally.

Your doctor should be able to refer you to a qualified practitioner of manipulation therapy in your area. For more information on accredited chiropractors, contact the American Chiropractic Association at (800) 986-4636, or online at www.amerchiro.org. For more information on licensed osteopaths, contact the American Osteopathic Association at (800) 621-1773, or online at www.aoc-net.org.

## MASSAGE

Massage is a common procedure used by many people who are not in chronic pain, but enjoy the soothing action of massage for stress relief or improvement in flexibility. But many people use massage for pain relief, and studies show that this is an effective, safe therapy when administered by a qualified professional. Massage therapists are plentiful and located in almost every area, and rates should be affordable.

Massage is a common term and there are several different types of massage. In a nutshell, massage is the manual manipulation and kneading of soft tissues, particularly muscles. Massage's benefits include improved blood circulation, relaxation of tense muscles, improved range of motion and increased endorphin levels – all of which may benefit people with chronic pain. Massage may enable you to feel more flexible and relaxed, so you sleep better and are more able to exercise regularly to maintain good health. Many doctors prescribe massage therapy to their chronic pain patients, and pain centers and clinics offer massage therapy as a key component of pain management.

Here's a rundown of the different types of massage therapy. Ask your doctor or physical therapist to suggest what type of massage is appropriate for your type of pain.

Swedish massage. This is the most common form of massage, and the form most people think of when they hear "massage." Swedish massage therapists knead the top layers of muscles of the body, often applying lotion or oil to ease their hand movements. Swedish massage usually lasts between 30 minutes and an hour. Some Swedish massage sessions are relaxing and others involve harder, more vigorous pressing designed to loosen tense muscles.

Deep tissue massage. This type of massage therapy involves a deeper, harder pressing by the therapist in order to release tension in the deepest layers of soft tissue. Therapists might use their fingers, elbows or thumbs to press between layers of muscles and get to the sources of pain or tension. Some people may experience soreness after the first few sessions, but later may find relief of nagging pain, such as low back pain or arthritis.

Trigger point therapy or neuromuscular massage. Trigger points are painful or tense points in the body that may be triggering pain elsewhere. In order to release the muscle tension that may be causing pain, practitioners use their fingers to press deeply into the body and massage those points. Some people with fibromyalgia find this therapy useful for tem-porary pain relief, but it can be a painful experience for others.

Myofascial release massage. Myofascial pain is centered in the fascia, or the fibrous, thin connective tissues beneath the skin, sheathing your muscles. In this massage therapy, practitioners gently massage and stretch the fascia in order to release tension in these structures. Typically, myofascial release therapy sessions last about 30 minutes, and don't use oil as in Swedish massage. People with myofascial pain, as well as fibromyalgia and pain caused by tension or stress, may find relief with this therapy.

Oriental massage techniques. As we discussed on p. 140, many Oriental medicine practitioners perform techniques designed to restore the flow of qi in the body. Acupressure is a massage-like technique where the practitioner presses on particular points of the body in an attempt to relieve pain that may occur in other areas of the body. According to the theory behind the therapy, these acupoints occur on energy pathways, or meridians, and the therapy is designed to restore proper energy flow and balance to relieve pain. *Shiatsu* massage is a Japanese technique that is gaining popularity in the West and is widely available at spas and health clubs where massage is offered. It's very similar to acupressure. Sessions may take place on a table or a mat on the floor, and include stretching techniques as well. A less widely practiced Oriental massage technique is *tuina,* a Chinese therapy that includes massaging the body's pressure points.

Rolfing. Rolfing (named for its inventor, Ida Rolf) involves a technique very similar to deep tissue massage, and the idea is that tightness in the fascia may be causing pain. Rolfing aims to release muscles and other soft tissues from the fascia so the body can restore its natural healing ability, aiming more at body maintenance than treating disease. Usually, Rolfing therapy takes place in 10 one-hour sessions held about a week apart. *Hellerwork* is a similar, massage-based practice that also involves exercises and teaching the person better posture and movement techniques in order to prevent pain.

Skinrolling technique. Some people with fibromyalgia find pain relief from this type of massage, although it is more widely used in Europe than in the United States. Skinrolling involves a therapist picking up a roll of the person's skin and moving it carefully back and forth across the fascia, the fibrous tissues underneath. This technique aims to break the connections between the tissue and the nerve endings under them that are communicating the pain messages. Skinrolling can be painful at first, so therapists may use a mild anesthetic before the treatment. Some people have reported long-lasting relief from fibromyalgia pain after skinrolling, but others find the technique itself too painful.

Spray and stretch technique. This kind of massage is used by people with fibromyalgia and also by people experiencing chronic back pain. Experts are divided on its validity. Spray and stretch is usually performed by a doctor or physical therapist rather than a massage therapist. The doctor or therapist sprays the skin over the painful area with a cooling anesthetic, such as flouri-methane, and then gently kneads the tense, painful muscles.

With any type of massage therapy, you should feel some relief after the session or at least in a few days. Most people who rely on massage therapy for pain relief schedule appointments regularly, as often as their doctor or physical therapist might suggest. But massage therapy can be expensive, so check your insurance policy carefully to see if the fees are covered if you have a doctor's prescription.

To find a qualified therapist, ask your doctor for a referral, or consult a physical therapy clinic or pain clinic or center in your area. If you use the services of a spa, make sure you check the credentials of the practitioners – they should be licensed massage therapists (LMTs). Be wary of so-called "massage parlors" or "health spas," which may offer cheaply priced massages performed by untrained, unlicensed people.

You can also perform your own massage to certain areas of the body that may be in pain, such as wrists, arms, legs, feet, neck or shoulders. It may be difficult for you to reach your own back, but you may be able to massage your own lower back. Massage devices are available at many retail stores. These devices can help you massage sore joints or muscles, and some can apply soothing heat as well.

## Reflexology

Similar to massage but more focused on a specific area of the body, *reflexology* is a pain-relief technique that is more similar to acupressure than traditional Swedish, full-body massage.

Reflexology practitioners believe that the hands, feet and ears have particular pressure points that correlate to completely different areas of the body or organs. When they apply pressure to these points, the correlating body part, which is in pain, will experience pain relief. For example, pressing on the heel might aid pain in the sciatic nerve, which is located in the back. Whether or not this theory is valid – and there are few studies to suggest that it is – some people may find the treatment soothing and relaxing. Others may experience the placebo effect and believe that the treatment will ease their pain.

## OTHER PAIN-RELIEF THERAPIES

There are numerous pain-relief therapies that either fall outside the standard medical treatment spectrum or are somewhat experimental. Many of these therapies are performed or prescribed by medical doctors and other mainstream health-care professionals, such as physical therapists. Before trying any of these therapies, talk to your doctor and consult your insurance coverage.

## TENS

Earlier in the book, we discussed implants that release electrical stimulation of nerves in order to relieve pain. (See p. 104.) Another type of electricity-based therapy is TENS, or transcutaneous electrical nerve stimulation. TENS uses electrical stimulation to the nerves to block pain signals from getting to the brain. Many doctors now suggest that their patients try this alternative pain treatment, especially people with back pain, arthritis, fibromyalgia or nerve-related pain. Doctors and other health-care professionals can administer TENS treatment to you.

TENS is not painful and requires no needles, surgery or drugs, so it's gaining in popularity as an alternative treatment for chronic pain. Usually, TENS helps people with pain concentrated in a particular area of the body, rather than all-over pain.

What Happens During TENS?  Your doctor or another practitioner will place small electrodes on your skin in the area where you are experiencing pain. He also attaches the electrodes to a small, battery-operated box that releases low-level electricity. When the box emits energy, you feel a low-level (but not painful) shock and a tingling feeling. If successful, TENS provides temporary pain relief.

TENS can be expensive, so it's not appropriate for everyone. In addition, people with widespread pain may not be able to use TENS. For some people, it offers short-term pain relief when other treatments fail to do so.

Ask your doctor to refer you to a TENS practitioner in your area. If there is a pain center or pain clinic in your area, the facility may be able to administer TENS. Inform your doctor if you decide to try TENS to make sure you are a good candidate.

## Biofeedback

As we learned in Chapter One, the brain is the control center for all pain messages. Your brain receives the pain signals from the nerves, "feels" the pain and decides how the body should respond. Can the brain also learn to control the way the body senses pain, perhaps reacting in a different way? An alternative treatment called *biofeedback* is based on the belief that it can.

Also called electromyography (EMG)-biofeedback, biofeedback involves a doctor, trained therapist or practitioner using electrical impulses to train you to try to control body functions – such as heart rate, blood pressure or body temperature – that normally are beyond your control. When people experience pain, they often become anxious and tense, feeling tightened muscles and an accelerated heartbeat that may make them feel worse. Biofeedback can help you respond to stress in a more positive way, and stress can cause or worsen pain.

Many hospitals, doctor's offices, pain centers, pain clinics and physical therapy offices offer biofeedback conducted by trained professionals. Ask your doctor to refer you to a qualified biofeedback practitioner if you want to explore this treatment.

**What happens during biofeedback?** In biofeedback, the doctor or therapist attaches electrodes or sensors to various parts of your body, particularly areas where you might be feeling pain or tension. The electrodes are connected to a computer or other instruments that record the various reactions you have to pain: body temperature, heart rate, muscle tension or even brain waves.

Then, you'll learn some mind-control techniques, such as visualization (focusing on pleasant imagery or fantasies where you are in control of your pain), or relaxation techniques, such as deep breathing. The practitioner will measure the impact these techniques have on your body's pain response. The biofeedback equipment should be able to show you how your relaxation techniques are affecting your body's processes. The practitioner will teach you to use these techniques to control your body's subconscious reactions. You'll have to do this several times and practice the techniques on your own. Eventually, you should be able to do these techniques on your own and see a positive result.

Does biofeedback really work? Some research shows that it can work, and learning relaxation therapies and seeing how they can affect your pain response is a positive, basically risk-free treatment option. You are learning to take control of your own body and your own reaction to pain. The NIH issued a consensus statement in 1995 stating that evidence shows that biofeedback can help people relieve many forms of chronic pain, such as back pain, and tension and migraine headaches.

## Hydrotherapy, Water Exercise and Balneotherapy

Better known as soaking in a hot tub, Jacuzzi™ or pool spa, *hydrotherapy* seems like a natural way to massage painful muscles and joints, or to relax the body in order to reduce painful muscle tension. You can explore hydrotherapy on your own, such as in your bathtub, hot tub or home whirlpool bath; at a health spa (in fact the word "spa" is an acronym for the Latin term *sante per aqua,* or "health by water"); or under medical supervision at a pain center, pain clinic or rehabilitation center.

The soothing but gentle pressure of water jets against sore, tightened or tense muscles can relieve back pain and other muscle-related pain. People with chronic pain syndromes that involve stress can find the soaking and bubbling action of the warm water relaxing. And soaking in warm or hot water is a widely recommended therapy for people with the joint pain and stiffness of arthritis. So hydrotherapy is an easy, low-risk therapy for many people in pain, something that may not completely relieve their pain but can be added as a complementary therapy to their pain-management plan. Hydrotherapy provides only temporary relief for chronic pain.

Some people cannot use hot tubs or spas, depending on their health condition. People with high blood pressure, diabetes or those taking some medicines should avoid hot tubs for health reasons. Ask your doctor if this therapy is acceptable for you and what, if any, precautions you should take. Do not mix alcohol or sedative drugs with hydrotherapy, as you could become drowsy and fall asleep in the water.

Another type of hydrotherapy is water exercise, a highly recommended and widely available therapy that is easy for most people with chronic pain to do. The Arthritis Foundation sponsors a water-exercise program, AFAP (Arthritis Foundation Aquatics Program), designed for people with arthritis, fibromyal-gia or any chronic pain syndrome. Exercises supervised by trained leaders and performed in warm pools allow the person to increase flexibility, cardiovascular health and muscle strength without the pain and strain of traditional land exercise. AFAP is also held at many YMCAs nationwide, where it's called AFYAP. Call the Arthritis Foundation at (800) 283-7800, or log on to www.arthritis.org, to find classes in your area.

A similar therapy that may provide warmth and relief to sore body parts is *balneotherapy,* or mud therapy. You may be familiar with mudpacks or herbal body wrap treatments at fancy spas as a way to relax the spirit. Some people also use warm mud compresses to relieve swelling and pain in joints.

A recent randomized, double-blind, controlled study conducted in Israel on people with rheumatoid arthritis affecting their hands showed possible promise for balneotherapy as a pain-relieving treatment. The doctors used compresses made of mineral-rich Dead Sea mud, a compound believed by some to have therapeutic effects on the body. Twenty-two of 45 patients received treatment with compresses of Dead Sea mud, while 23 others received mud depleted of minerals. The patients who used the mineral-rich mudpacks saw greater improvement in their symptoms than the group who used mineral-depleted mud, including reduction in the number of tender or swollen joints and a reduction in their perception of pain severity.

While more research is needed to determine if the mineral content of the mud, the mud itself, or just the soothing warmth of the mud compresses helps people's painful joints feel better, this therapy may provide some temporary relief of pain or, at least, relaxation.

## Hypnosis

Many people associate hypnosis with carnival entertainment or trickery. But this serious, widespread treatment dates back a few hundred years, and is utilized by many medical professionals. Hypnosis may be effective for some people in chronic pain, according to several published studies. While some people can hypnotize themselves, it may be easier at first to work with a trained professional, such as a psychiatrist, licensed psychologist or therapist.

Hypnosis was first used by Franz Anton Mesmer, an Austrian physician, who used it to treat patients with various nervous conditions or ailments by lulling them into a state of extreme mental relaxation. This practice, first known as *mesmerism* after its creator, involved the person staring at a light or object until they reached this very relaxed state.

Hypnosis is done much the same way today. In this state, the person is more susceptible to suggestion, and the doctor could help the person learn to relax tense muscles or reduce the stress that may be causing or worsening pain. Hypnosis has been used as a therapy for chronic migraine headaches, as well as other painful conditions.

## Ultrasound Therapy

Ultrasound or ultrasonography (see p. 40) sometimes is used in diagnosis. It also may be used as a therapy: The high-frequency sounds waves emit a soothing heat that may be used to relieve muscle or tissue pain. Similar to the heat therapy provided by heating pads or even hydrotherapy, ultrasound offers only temporary relief.

Ultrasound therapy equipment is not available to the public. A health-care professional (usually a physical therapist) trained in ultrasound must administer the therapy. So repeated treatments can be expensive and time-consuming. Doctors usually prescribe ultrasound therapy only when a person is experiencing a severe flare of pain that may not be adequately relieved by pain medicines. Ultrasound therapy is not recommended for people whose pain is accompanied by inflammation, because the heat might worsen the swelling. But for many people, ultrasound therapy is a useful complement to their pain-management treatments.

A similar type of ultrasound therapy called *shock-wave therapy* was not found to be very beneficial in a recent Australian study, where people with the painful foot condition plantar fasciitis underwent treatment of shock or sound waves over a three-week period. Plantar fasciitis is also known as a heel spur, and involves painful inflammation of the connective tissue on the bottom of the foot. The shock-wave therapy aimed to break up scar tissue and stimulate blood circulation to promote healing, but the treatment didn't work any better than a placebo treatment. However, as with many complementary therapies, you may find some relief with ultrasound.

Consult your doctor to see if he recommends using this therapy for your pain condition.

## Prolotherapy

A relatively new experimental technique for chronic pain relief, *prolotherapy* aims to relieve pain by rebuilding and strengthening weakened connective tissues, particularly ligaments and tendons that may be painful due to injury or continued stress or pressure. Because muscles, ligaments and tendons support the bones, when they weaken you are more susceptible to pain and further injury.

Prolotherapy is often used to treat back pain, neck pain, sciatica or *whiplash*, a common and painful condition where the neck is whipped back and forth suddenly due to an impact, such as a car accident. Prolotherapy is also called sclerotherapy, proliferative injection therapy, stimulated ligament repair, regenerative injection therapy or nonsurgical ligament reconstruction. As these names suggest, the therapy is meant to repair or restore the damaged or weakened connective tissues that can no longer properly support joints and bones, leading to pain with every movement. Doctors usually administer prolotherapy.

Prolotherapy differs from other injection therapies, and that's why it's still controversial and not supported by some doctors. In prolotherapy, the doctor injects an irritating solution into the damaged or painful soft tissues. Rather than traditional injections, which use an anti-inflammatory medication, prolotherapy's aim is to create inflammation. Why? Proponents of the therapy believe this intentional inflammation will increase blood circulation in the painful area and hasten the healing process. So the small tears or weaknesses in the damaged connective tissues will heal, the tissues will strengthen and the pain will subside. Normally, the process takes about four to six weeks.

Prolotherapy is still controversial because most doctors abide by a philosophy of "do no harm," and the therapy intentionally creates inflammation – a condition most doctors wish to heal. More and more doctors and pain centers are performing prolotherapy, so ask your doctor about this procedure.

## Aromatherapy

Sniffing pleasant fragrances is a soothing, relaxing activity, but some people have refined this practice into a treatment called *aromatherapy*. Aromatherapy involves smelling various fragrances from essential oils (concentrated amounts of a certain fragrance), candles or incense to relax, relieve pain and reduce symptoms. Popular aromatherapy essential oils include eucalyptus, peppermint, rosemary, laurel, chamomile, marjoram, jasmine and lavender. Epsom salts or sea salts may be used in hot aromatherapy baths.

Use of aromatic herbs or incense as a way to heal physical or emotional pain dates back thousands of years. The ancient Egyptians, Chinese, Greeks, Indians and other civilizations used such practices as part of their healing rites. During the Black Death epidemic in medieval Europe, doctors felt that pestilence and disease might spread in foul-smelling air or mists, leading to a practice of wearing masks containing fragrance as a way to purify the air they breathed and protect them from disease.

In 1928, a French practitioner named Rene Maurice Gattefosse coined the term "aromatherapy" to describe the emerging contemporary practice of using fragrance for healing. Aromatherapy has gained popularity in the last ten years as a method of relieving stress and healing various problems. However, the term may be misunderstood, applied too broadly or misused. Many product manufacturers use the term aromatherapy to promote any good-smelling product, from candles to room sprays to carpet deodorizers.

Aromatherapy as a pain-relief therapy involves smelling specific scents for certain purposes. You can be aided by an aromatherapy practitioner or therapist, who will administer the treatments or guide you in doing it yourself. Aromatherapy applications include massage with particular oils, steam baths with essential oils added to the steam source, aromatic baths to soak in, inhalation using a cloth or an electronic diffuser, candles, sprays, aromatic rubs or creams and more.

Aromatherapy may not provide effective relief for chronic pain, but some aromatherapy treatments may provide relaxation, easing tense muscles. Hot baths or steam baths might be soothing to sore joints and muscles, and adding the essential oil may provide some additional soothing qualities to the mind. It is important to use any of these treatments properly and with the knowledge of your doctor. Some essential oils or creams that come in

contact with the skin might cause rashes or other skin irritations. It's important to keep any essential oils or other fragrance sources away from the eyes, particularly sprays that might contain alcohol, chemical propellants or other irritants.

Does aromatherapy really work? Evidence does not yet support the efficacy of this therapy on its own for pain relief, but aromatherapy may provide help in achieving relaxation, leading to easing of tense muscles that can cause pain.

## CONTROVERSIAL ALTERNATIVE THERAPIES

Some other alternative treatments for chronic pain are controversial and spark a division of opinion and debate among doctors and other health-care professionals. Many of these treatments simply may not work, or they may work for some people but not for others. Some people feel that if something can't hurt, it's worth trying. That's up to you: Most therapies require some cost as well as your time and effort. So saying "it couldn't hurt" is really not true. If you pay for something that doesn't work and can't easily get a refund for your money, it hurts! You also may feel discouraged by the failed treatment, causing additional stress and anxiety about your chronic pain.

The best way to avoid this situation is to consult your doctor for advice. You can also conduct some of your own research on the Internet or by reading reputable health journals for reports of study results on various treatments. The Arthritis Foundation Web site posts the latest news of medical study results on treatments for chronic pain, including alternative therapies, as do many other medical organizations. Consult these sources for trustworthy, objective information.

Here are a few other treatments for chronic pain that could be considered controversial:

Low-powered lasers. Lasers, beams of highly concentrated light, first appeared in science-fiction movies, but some doctors and physical therapists zap painful areas of the body with low-powered laser beams as a way to stimulate cell growth, boost endorphin production, treat inflammation or promote healing of damaged nerves. Lasers are also used successfully in some surgeries. But it remains unproven if this therapy really works for treating chronic pain.

Magnet therapy. The wearing or application of magnets as a method of healing or pain relief is ancient, first used by the Egyptians and Greeks. Modern people in pain revived the practice in recent years as a way to relieve pain, particularly after injuries, accidents, or in cases of arthritis, fibromyalgia or back pain. Magnets are usually worn as a wristband or neck collar.

The therapy aims to change the way cells behave or to alter body chemistry to promote healing, but many doctors, scientists and skeptics claim this treatment is pure bunk – just a ploy to get you to buy a magnet bracelet or device. However, magnetic therapy may hold some promise after more studies are conducted. Many magnets sold in retail stores or through the Internet have no power and prob-

ably no benefit, but the future of magnet therapy may lie in more powerful devices that can emit a stronger form of magnetic energy, called pulse electromagnetic therapy. This therapy, rising in popularity, may be more worthwhile.

Gin-soaked raisins. Soaking raisins in gin or other alcoholic beverages and eating them is an old folk remedy for arthritis pain. The gin may offer a temporary dulling of aches, but alcohol is not recommended as a pain reliever. While it may be tasty, gin-soaked raisins do not offer any real medical benefit.

Marijuana. Marijuana, the common name for the widely grown but illegally (in most countries) sold or used plant *cannabis sativa,* is highly controversial as an analgesic and anti-nausea treatment. Many battles between the legal, political, medical and patient communities are taking place as some people in chronic pain fight for the option to use marijuana as a medicine. Marijuana, when smoked or ingested, can create an extreme sense of relaxation and pain relief for a time. Yet it can also be psychologically addictive, and is viewed negatively as a street drug.

Some studies show that marijuana may have a positive effect on pain receptors in the brain and help to reduce the brain's pain response, similar to the way analgesic drugs work. Some scientists are trying to isolate the actual chemical in the marijuana that has this benefit, so they can develop a pill form that doesn't cause the "high" that sparks such controversy. In some areas, some patients can receive "medical marijuana" under very controlled circumstances. These people are usually cancer or AIDS patients. More studies are required to determine if a medical use for marijuana in terms of chronic pain treatment merit legalization as a controlled substance that can be prescribed by doctors.

Whether or not you wish to try an alternative treatment for your pain or just stick to more tried-and-true options, there are an increasing number of treatments available to explore. Some of these treatments are less involved or invasive than others, allowing you to try them without significant risk or cost. It's important to be informed before you try any alternative or complementary treatment, and to tell your doctor whatever you do. In some cases, your doctor can offer you a referral or suggestions about what treatments will work best for your type of pain, and many doctors are open to their patients creating an integrative pain-management plan.

Some treatments that lie outside the realm of drugs or surgery, but are not quite as experimental as those covered in this chapter, are what we call "do-it-yourself" therapies or lifestyle management techniques. A person in chronic pain needs to create a healthy overall lifestyle to control their daily pain and to manage the underlying disease that causes the pain.

This concept is at the heart of any successful pain-management plan. You likely will hear your doctor tell you that pain medicines won't do the job alone – your actions are also an incredibly powerful weapon in the fight against chronic pain. Exercise, proper diet, relaxation and stress management, learning proper movement and getting proper sleep will help your body heal injuries, restore energy, increase flexibility and even lessen pain. While exercising may be the last thing you want to do when you're in pain, it might be the first thing you should do each day to prevent and lessen pain.

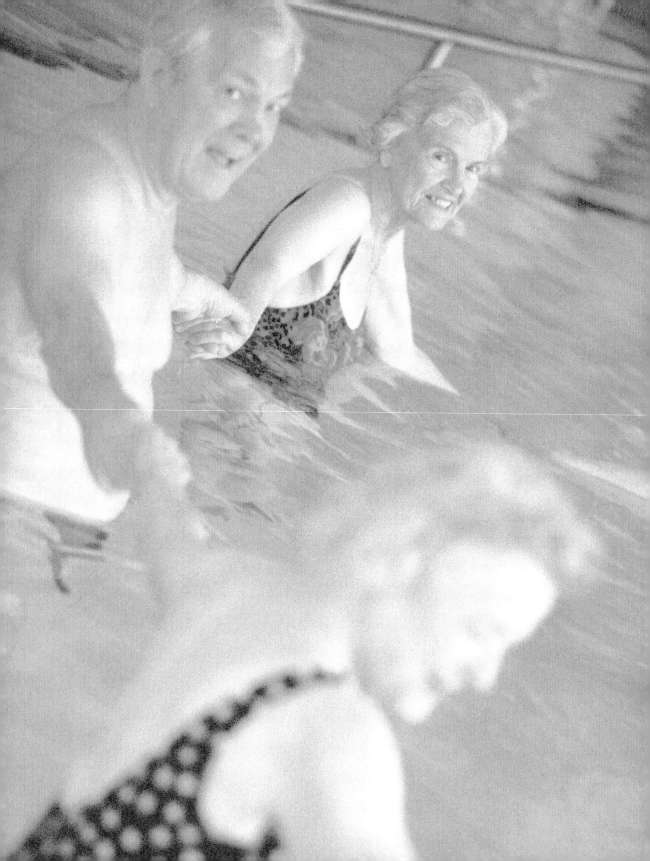

# Do-It-Yourself Pain Relief

9

# CHAPTER 9: DO-IT-YOURSELF PAIN RELIEF

At the heart of every pain-management plan are not only the treatments your doctor offers – including drugs, surgery or special pain-relief therapies – but also what you can do on your own to control chronic pain and boost general health.

Many alternative treatments seek to restore the body's natural ability to heal itself. While these therapies may or may not be scientifically valid, there is something basic and true in the idea behind them. When your body is working as well as it can through proper diet, exercise and stress management, it can better deal with chronic pain conditions. Muscles that are toned can better support joints weakened by arthritis. Ligaments and tendons that are flexible can promote easier, less painful movement. A mind that does not suffer from oppressive stress can promote better sleep and more relaxed muscles.

Not every pain-relief technique involves drugs or surgery, doctors or practitioners. There are many things you can do at home to provide temporary, but often noticeable, pain relief, techniques that don't cost much and can be done easily at any time. In addition, there are many methods you can try to reduce stress without having to rely on a doctor or therapist's help, although you may need professional help if your stress becomes too much for you to control on your own.

In addition to your doctor, there are health-care professionals who can help guide you in do-it-yourself pain relief and pain prevention methods. Physical therapists can help you create a plan of exercise tailored to your physical needs and limitations. Occupational therapists can help you adjust the way you perform various activities, particularly at your job, to reduce pain and prevent injury. In addition, these professionals can prescribe braces, splints and other aids for you that may reduce pain while you are experiencing a flare or healing from an injury. Braces and splints can be very effective, temporary help in relieving unusual episodes of pain.

First, let's discuss some easy pain-relief techniques that you can do at home. Then, we'll look at some basic principles of exercise for pain management, and diet for good health. In the next chapter, we'll go over some methods you can try to reduce or control stress to keep it from worsening your pain.

## THE POWER OF HEAT AND COLD

Two of the simplest, least expensive and most effective methods of pain relief are heat and cold treatments. Heat treatments, such as heating pads or warm baths, tend to work best for soothing stiff joints and painful muscles due to arthritis, fibromyalgia or back pain.

Heat helps your body get limber and ready for exercise or activity. Cold treatments work best for flares of pain, numbing the area and decreasing inflammation. Try different forms of heat and cold therapy and see what works best for you.

## Heat Treatments

Here are some useful tips for applying heat for pain relief.

- Take a long, very warm shower first thing in the morning to ease morning stiffness, or a warm shower when you have a painful flare. Use the water jet to massage a specific, sore area, such as your lower back.
- Try thermal wraps available in most pharmacies and supermarkets. These items, which provide low-level heat over an 8-hour period, do not need to be heated in a microwave oven.
- Try warm paraffin wax treatment systems, available at many drugstores or beauty supply stores. Dip arms, wrists, hand and feet into the soothing heat.
- Soak in a warm bath, hot tub or spa. Try positioning the painful area in front of the water jets for massage.
- Use a moist heating pad or make one at home by putting a wet washcloth in a freezer bag and heating it in the microwave for 1 minute. Wrap the hot pack in a towel and place it over the affected area for 15 to 20 minutes.
- Rub mineral oil on painful hands, slip on rubber dishwashing gloves and place your hands in hot tap water for 5 to 10 minutes.
- Warm your clothes in the dryer before dressing each day.
- Use an electric blanket and turn it up for a few minutes before getting out of bed.

## Cold Treatments

Here are some useful tips for applying cold for pain relief.

- Wrap a bag of ice in a towel and apply it to sore joints for about 10 minutes.

## HEAT AND COLD: BE SAFE!

When using heat and cold pain therapies, avoid burns by following these guidelines:

- Use the heat or cold therapy for no more than 15 to 20 minutes at a time. Let your skin return to normal temperature before reapplying heat or cold.
- Don't place an ice or heat pack or pad directly on your skin — always use a towel or cloth in between.
- Never use analgesic creams, ointments or gels at the same time as heat treatments, as you can cause serious skin burns.
- Don't sleep with an electric heating pad on. This is a fire hazard and can also lead to excessive heating of your skin and tissues.
- Be careful using heat patches or heating pads on parts of the body that may be desensitized, such as in diabetes or other health conditions. You risk serious burns.

- Try cooling (containing menthol, oil of wintergreen or other cooling agents) topical creams on sore joints and muscles.
- Use a gel-filled cold pack from the drugstore and apply it to painful areas for about 10 minutes.
- Wrap a towel around a bag of frozen vegetables and place it on painful joints. This type of cold pack easily conforms to your joints.
- Use one of these cold treatments following exercise to soothe any sore joints or muscles.

## Self-Massage

Massage given by a trained therapist can provide good pain relief, but you can also administer your own massage to sore areas of your body. Your doctor, physical therapist or massage therapist can show you some techniques to use at home.

You can simply knead sore areas with your hands, but there are many self-massage appliances that can help you massage hard-to-reach places of the body. In addition, some people with painful hands or fingers may find it difficult to do self-massage without the assistance of a massage aid device.

Massage aids come in all styles and price ranges. There are a wide variety of non-electric massage aids that have rolling rubber or wooden balls on ropes or hand-held wands for under $20. Electric hand-held massagers, which have vibrating balls or knobs that knead sore muscles, range in price from $14 to $150. These come in many different styles and shapes, and may be battery-operated or plugged into an electrical outlet. Foot massage units, which can

also contain warm water, can cost from $25 to $400. There are car seat covers that heat up and massage your back, buttocks and thighs while driving. These items cost around $130. Full-body massage chairs can cost in the thousands.

Use these tips before self-massage to make the experience easier and more effective.

- Take a warm bath or shower first to relax your muscles, improve blood circulation and make your hands and fingers more limber.
- Use oil or lotion to help your hands glide over sore areas.
- Use a tennis ball or other soft rubber ball to help massage the back, buttocks, thighs or other sore areas. You can lie down, place the ball beneath the sore spot and roll against it on the floor or on a firm mattress.

## Joint Protection

One of the best things you can do to prevent flares of pain or injuries that will worsen pain is to protect the areas of your body that are in pain. As you move during the course of each day, your sore, damaged joints may become stressed. We put pressure on our joints, muscles and other tissues each time we walk, lift, carry, bend down, climb stairs, twist with our hands, cut, write, reach up or do almost any other activity. You can learn ways to protect your sore joints to avoid undue pressure and further injury.

It's important to keep moving so your body doesn't become weak and more susceptible to pain. Don't avoid activity, just use some creativity!

Here are a few things to remember:

- **Consider joint position.** Use joints in the best way to avoid excess stress. Use larger, stronger joints such as your arms and legs to push or carry. For example, if you have to carry a load of groceries into the house, hug the bag with your arms and hold it close to your body so you can support the load better. Don't grip the edges of the bag or the handle with your fingers. If you have to move a large object, see if you can push it with your lower body instead of trying to pull it with your hands.

- **Use helpful devices.** There are numerous appliances available to help you grab, reach, pull, push and move around. Not just canes, crutches and walkers, but also grips to add to pens so you can hold them with less finger stress, long-handled reachers to help you grasp items that sit high or low, and attachments to door knobs or car door handles to help you open and close doors. Use devices to help you open containers like flip-top cans and jars. Select light-weight tools and appliances. Look for products designed for ease of use or make your own (such as attaching a foam-rubber hair curler to a toothbrush for easier gripping).

- **Put it on wheels.** If you have to move things from room to room, such as heavy files, laundry or gardening supplies, use a child's red wagon, a rolling cart or a suitcase with wheels and a pull-up handle.

- **Ask for help if you need it.** Don't be afraid to ask family, friends or coworkers for help doing a task. Don't risk injury to your body just because you're afraid of hurting your pride.

## EXERCISE: BOOST THE BODY'S DEFENSES

As we said at the end of the last chapter, when you are in pain on a daily basis, the first thing you may want to do is skip your exercise routine. Who wants to work out when your body hurts? Sometimes you may feel as if you can't even get off the couch, much less get on a treadmill or take a walk. While rest is important for people with chronic pain, so is exercise and movement.

The second thing you may discard is your healthy diet. When you're in pain and stressed out from the pain, you may want comfort food that is easy to prepare, like frozen pizzas or take-out Chinese noodles. But this type of diet – high in sodium, fat and calories and low in nutrients – can sap your body of energy and lessen its ability to recharge and heal. Without the healthiest body possible (although we realize you have chronic pain), you may be less able to handle medications or surgical procedures designed to treat your pain, leading to debilitating side effects, fatigue or lengthy recoveries after procedures. Your pain may only grow worse.

When you have chronic pain, it's important to commit to making regular exercise and a healthy diet the cornerstone of your pain-management plan. These healthy practices, along with your medications and other treatments your doctor prescribes, can help you fight your chronic pain on a number of fronts. Pain may be caused by disease or injury, but you can more easily fight the disease, heal the injury and control the pain when you are in the best physical and emotional shape possible.

## The Benefits of Exercise for Pain

If you are in pain, it can be difficult to get up and move around. You hurt, so you don't feel like moving. You feel like resting on the couch, not riding a bike or lifting weights. So you give up exercise, and after a short period of time, your body deteriorates. You lose some flexibility or range of motion. Your muscles, unused and dormant, may weaken or *atrophy,* making them more painful and less able to support weakened joints if you have arthritis. Your tendons, ligaments and other connective tissues, since you are not flexing and stretching them regularly, become less flexible and more susceptible to painful tearing, strain and inflammation. Your bones, because you are not performing important weight-bearing exercises (like walking or lifting weights), may weaken, leading to osteoporosis. People with osteoporosis are more susceptible to painful, debilitating fractures and dangerous falls.

As you can see, not exercising is a terrible break in your body's cycle of good health, making chronic pain worse and lessening your ability to fight painful conditions and diseases.

OK, you know the downside of not exercising. Why will exercise help you fight chronic pain? Exercise has many proven, pain-fighting benefits. Regular exercise that contains the three basic types of movement – cardiovascular or heart-revving exercise, flexibility or range-of-motion exercises, and strengthening or muscle-and-bone-building exercise – can improve your heart and blood circulation, build stronger bones, and increase flexibility to reduce strains of soft tissues. Exercise also boosts your brain's natural production of endorphins, those pain-fighting hormones that act much the same as analgesic medicines. Exercise also can reduce stress and anxiety, which can worsen pain or even cause painful muscle tension. Exercise can help.

Exercise also can burn calories to help you lose weight or control weight. This is an important benefit because excess pounds on your frame can add great stress to bones, joints, nerves and muscles that may be damaged or weakened due to your chronic disease. People who weigh the appropriate amount for their age, height and body style often experience less pain than those who are overweight or *obese,* extremely overweight. People who are overweight may have more difficult surgery or recovery.

## A Solid Exercise Plan

What is a good exercise program that will help you manage your chronic pain? For one, you should exercise regularly – at least three to five times per week, and at least 30 minutes to an hour per session. Don't worry if you do not exercise now – you can work up to this level slowly. In fact, most doctors or physical therapists would not recommend that you go from doing no exercise to trying to jog three miles a day. You would only fail to complete your run, probably hurt yourself and likely never want to exercise again! Start with a gentle, regular exercise routine and slowly add different components to create a comprehensive plan.

That plan should include exercises that fall into these three categories:

- **Flexibility or range-of-motion exercises:** When you stretch, bend or sway to increase mobility of joints.
- **Strengthening or weight-bearing exercises:** When you apply force to body resistance. Lifting weights and movements that involve resistance of the body fall in this category.
- **Cardiovascular, aerobic or endurance exercises:** When you move large muscles at a sustained rate over a period of time, increasing your heart rate and working up a sweat. Aerobic exercise strengthens the heart, circulatory system and lungs, and includes dancing, fast walking, swimming and jogging.

All types of exercise serve to reduce stress, so if your plan starts with just one or two of the three components, you should see some stress-relief benefit. And that's good for controlling pain. As you build your exercise program to include more techniques and longer time spent exercising, your pain-control and stress-management benefits will only increase.

## Can Exercise Increase My Pain?

You may fear exercise because you think you will worsen your pain or damage your muscles and joints. This is understandable. Warming up with stretching before you exercise, and cooling down with more stretching and breathing after you exercise, will help you avoid injury or pain due to exercise.

It's important to learn the difference between the type of pain you experience from sore muscles after exercising and the type of pain caused by overuse or inflammation of joints. Sore muscles usually stem from overstretching or overusing muscles by working out after a long period of not exercising at all. This type of pain normally begins several hours after your workout and may continue for 24 to 36 hours.

If you do have exercise-related muscle pain, increase your warm-up exercises before proceeding to the rest of your exercise activity, or scale back your program until your muscles become more accustomed to exercise. Once you feel that you are used to your program, gradually increase the length and/or intensity of your workout.

When you overuse joints by exercise, usually you experience pain or swelling. If you notice these symptoms (see the box on p. 164), treat the problem by elevating the effected area, resting it and using ice packs to lessen swelling. Talk to your doctor or therapist about your exercise program and the problems you encountered.

Some people with chronic pain may not be able to perform some exercises, but should be able to find techniques that fall into all of the above categories. Some exercises are jarring to bones and joints, or involve extreme bending or stretching that may be too painful or difficult for your condition. Don't worry! You can achieve the same benefits from less strenuous techniques.

## ARE YOU DOING TOO MUCH?

As we said earlier in this chapter, if you don't exercise at all, start slowly as you begin working out. Increase your activity level at a gradual pace to avoid injuries or more pain – not something you want if you already have a chronic pain condition.

Look for these signs that you may be overexerting yourself:

• Increased or unusual pain that lasts for more than an hour after exercise

• Increased feelings of weakness
• Excessive fatigue after exercise
• Decreased range of motion or flexibility

If you experience these feelings, cut back on the amount of time you spend exercising or on the level of exertion, and call your doctor or physical therapist. He or she may be able to suggest a change in your routine as well as a temporary pain-relief measure for your exercise-related pain.

---

No matter what your situation, you should consult your doctor before beginning any exercise program. Talk to him about your problems and needs. He should be able to suggest a beneficial and manageable exercise program for you, or can refer you to a physical therapist or exercise specialist who can guide you in your workouts. If your doctor does not provide a referral, ask for one or consult a licensed physical therapist on your own. These professionals can help you find the right exercise for your ability level and pain condition. Inform any therapist about your diagnosis right away so your limitations or challenges are clear from the start.

Luckily, there are many easy and gentle exercises that you can do to begin increasing flexibility, cardiovascular health and strength, exercises that don't involve expensive club memberships, fancy equipment or a big chunk of your daily free time. In addition, there are many alternative forms of exercise that involve less sweat and strain than the traditional "workout," but achieve many pain-management benefits. We'll go over some of the best pain-management exercise routines here, and also offer some gentle stretching exercises anyone can do to increase flexibility.

### Flexibility Exercises

When you have chronic pain, you might hate to move any more than necessary. It is very important to stay mobile, moving all your joints through their range of motion on a regular basis. Each joint has a range of motion, which is the fullest extent you can move it in any direction. If you don't keep joints flexible through proper exercise, you could experience stiffness, immobility and more pain. Maintaining range of motion is key to having the best quality of life you can.

Flexibility or range-of-motion exercises are daily stretches designed to help you keep joints limber and mobile even if you have chronic pain. You can incorporate these stretches into your normal routine. For example, perform them in the morning after your morning shower or bath and before you get dressed for the day. Do range-of-motion stretches before any activity that may be exerting, such as a shopping trip or attending the office picnic, to keep your body limber. Limber muscles and joints can help you maintain balance, avoid falls and prevent injuries or aches. You can do flexibility stretches almost anywhere, even in a pool or hot tub.

Tips: Use gentle, smooth movements rather than quickly jerking your limbs, neck and other movable parts. Wear clothes that allow you to move your joints through their full range of motion with ease. Choose a place that is comfortable and gives you enough room to stretch your limbs fully.

The Arthritis Foundation chapter office nearest you will have information about exercise classes that are safe for people with chronic pain. These classes include the Arthritis Foundation Aquatics Program (also taught at many YMCA pools) and PACE, or People with Arthritis Can Exercise, a program of easy exercises for people with impaired mobility. These courses are also available on videotape. See the Resources section of this book for more information.

EXERCISE 2: SHOULDER CIRCLES

- MOVE SHOULDERS SLOWLY IN A CIRCULAR MOTION.

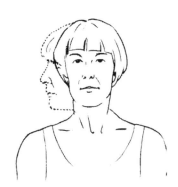

EXERCISE 1: HEAD TURNS

- LOOK STRAIGHT AHEAD.
- TURN HEAD TO LOOK OVER SHOULDER.
- HOLD THREE SECONDS.
- RETURN TO FRONT.
- REPEAT ON THE OTHER SIDE.

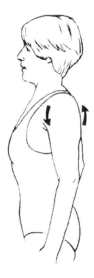

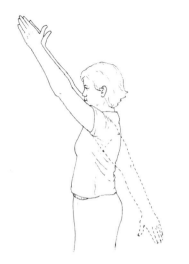

EXERCISE 3: FORWARD ARM REACH

- POSITION YOUR ARMS OUT IN FRONT, PALMS FACING
  ONE ANOTHER.
- RAISE ONE OR BOTH ARMS FORWARD AND UP AS
  HIGH AS POSSIBLE (ONE ARM MAY HELP THE OTHER,
  IF NEEDED).
- LOWER ARMS SLOWLY.

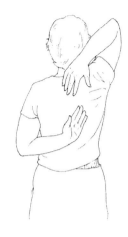

EXERCISE 4: BACK PAT AND RUB

- REACH ONE ARM UP TO PAT BACK.
- REACH THE OTHER ARM BEHIND YOUR LOWER BACK.
- SLIDE HANDS TOWARD EACH OTHER.
- HOLD THREE SECONDS.
- ALTERNATE ARM POSITION.

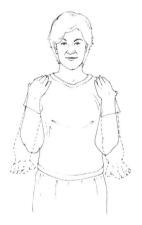

EXERCISE 5: ELBOW BEND AND TURN

TOUCH FINGERS TO SHOULDERS, PALMS TOWARD YOU.
TURN PALMS DOWN AS YOU STRAIGHTEN ELBOWS OUT
TO SIDE.

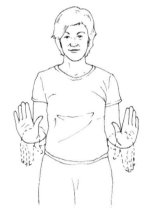

EXERCISE 6: WRIST BEND

- STAND WITH ELBOWS TUCKED TO SIDES.
- BEND WRISTS UP.
- HOLD THREE SECONDS.
- BEND WRISTS DOWN.
- HOLD THREE SECONDS.

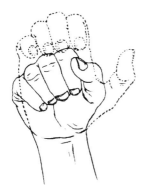

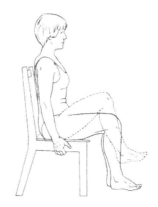

EXERCISE 7: FINGER CURL

- OPEN HAND FLAT, FINGERS STRAIGHT.
- BEND EACH JOINT SLOWLY TO MAKE A LOOSE FIST.
- HOLD THREE SECONDS.
- STRAIGHTEN FINGERS AGAIN.

EXERCISE 8: KNEE LIFT

- SIT STRAIGHT UP IN A CHAIR.
- LIFT ONE KNEE UP THREE OR FOUR INCHES OFF CHAIR.
- HOLD THREE SECONDS AND LOWER.
- REPEAT WITH OTHER KNEE (YOU MAY HELP BY LIFTING THE KNEE WITH YOUR HANDS UNDER YOUR THIGH).

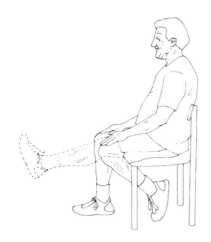

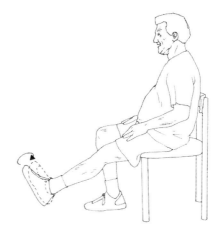

EXERCISE 9: LEG BEND AND LIFT

- SIT UP STRAIGHT IN A CHAIR.
- BEND KNEE, PUTTING YOUR HEEL UNDER THE CHAIR.
- HOLD THREE SECONDS.
- STRAIGHTEN KNEE OUT IN FRONT.
- HOLD THREE SECONDS.

EXERCISE 10: ANKLE CIRCLES

- CURL TOES DOWN.
- HOLD THREE SECONDS.
- LIFT TOES UP.
- HOLD THREE SECONDS.

VARIATIONS: PICK UP A TOWEL OR SOME MARBLES WITH YOUR TOES.

## Strengthening Exercises

There are many ways to build strength in your muscles and improve the condition of your bones, tendons and ligaments. Strengthening exercises that build muscle tone will help keep your joints stable and make movement easier. Weight training is a logical method that comes to mind as a way to build strength, but this method may not be a good choice for you if you don't exercise at all or find weightlifting intimidating. You can build strength slowly and easily through simple exercises, even moves you can do while sitting in a chair.

Two common strengthening exercises that are good for people in chronic pain are isometric exercises and isotonic exercises. In isometric exercises, you tense or tighten muscles, but don't move joints. In isotonic exercises, you concentrate on moving joints. Isotonic exercises are different from simple stretching or range-of-motion exercises (see p. 164). They emphasize building muscle strength. Here are sample exercises in each category:

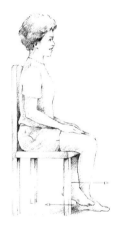

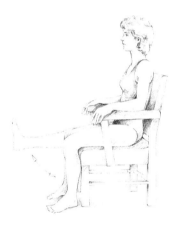

ISOMETRIC EXERCISE:

SIT IN A STRAIGHT-BACKED CHAIR AND CROSS YOUR ANKLES. YOUR LEGS CAN BE ALMOST STRAIGHT, OR YOU CAN BEND YOUR KNEES AS MUCH AS YOU LIKE. PUSH FORWARD WITH YOUR BACK LEG AND PRESS BACKWARD WITH YOUR FRONT LEG. EXERT PRESSURE EVENLY SO THAT YOUR LEGS DO NOT MOVE. HOLD AND COUNT OUT LOUD FOR SIX TO 10 SECONDS. RELAX. THEN CHANGE LEG POSITIONS AND REPEAT.

AS YOU DO THIS EXERCISE REGULARLY, YOU CAN ADD REPETITIONS (THE AMOUNT OF TIMES YOU DO THE MOVE) TO BUILD MORE STRENGTH.

ISOTONIC EXERCISE:

SIT IN A CHAIR WITH BOTH FEET ON THE FLOOR AND SPREAD SLIGHTLY APART. RAISE ONE FOOT UNTIL YOUR LEG IS AS STRAIGHT AS YOU CAN MAKE IT. HOLD AND COUNT OUT LOUD FOR SIX TO 10 SECONDS. GENTLY LOWER YOUR FOOT TO THE FLOOR. RELAX. REPEAT WITH THE OTHER LEG.

AS YOU DO THIS EXERCISE REGULARLY, YOU CAN ADD REPETITIONS OR USE LIGHT ANKLE WEIGHTS (1-2 POUNDS TO START) TO INCREASE RESISTANCE.

Weight training. While lifting weights may seem like an activity favored more by young, muscle-bound men than people with chronic pain, you may be surprised to see more and more older adults lifting at your local gym. Weight training, whether with free weights (such as bar bells or dumb bells), weight machines or weighted ankle and wrist straps, is a good way to build muscle strength and tone, and increase bone density. It can also help control your weight and burn calories.

Do not lift weights without first consulting your doctor and then, work out with the supervision of a qualified exercise specialist. It's important to start with a small amount of weight and gradually build up what you lift to prevent injury. As you build strength, you also can increase repetitions.

## Cardiovascular or Aerobic Exercise

You know you are "working out" when you break a sweat and feel your heart pumping a little bit. Those are two signs that you are doing aerobic or cardiovascular exercise, which is great for maintaining good circulation, a healthy heart and proper body weight.

While most people hear the word "aerobics" and think of people jumping around a gymnasium floor dressed in skimpy outfits, there are many gentle, easy forms of aerobic exercise. Cardiovascular exercise can include many different activities. This type of exercise should involve you moving large muscles (such as your legs) in a continuous, rhythmic movement (such as in walking) for a period of time long enough to raise your heart rate. The new government guidelines suggest an hour a day of aerobic exercise, although it can be divided into chunks for convenience. Doing aerobic exercises regularly will build your stamina, making it easier to do other activities with less fatigue.

Here are some fun, easy aerobic exercises you can try on your own. Be willing to experiment so your exercise routine does not become a boring routine!

Walking. Walking is arguably the cheapest, easiest, most convenient form of exercise, because you can do it almost anywhere or anytime. Walking is an excellent type of cardiovascular and calorie-burning exercise for almost anyone. Walking requires no special skills except the ability to walk.

To walk regularly for exercise, you do need a safe, convenient place to walk. It may be helpful and safer to walk with a spouse, friend or a group of neighbors. You can walk almost anytime and anywhere. Many areas have mall-walking clubs. You should have supportive walking shoes and comfortable clothes. Shoes that are uncomfortable or not suitable for walking can actually increase your pain. See p. 171 for a walking plan.

Water Exercise. As we mentioned in the previous chapter, water exercise can be good for stiff, painful joints and sore muscles that are common for people with chronic pain conditions. Warm water supports your body while you move your joints through their range of

## HELPFUL WALKING RESOURCES

If you need some motivation or guidance as you begin walking for fitness, the Arthritis Foundation has a nationwide program called *Walk With Ease*. Your local Arthritis Foundation chapter will have more information on how you can get involved in a walking club in your neighborhood or start your own.

The Arthritis Foundation publishes a guide to walking for exercise if you have chronic pain called *Walk With Ease: Your Guide to Walking for Better Health, Improved Fitness and Less Pain*. The book, as well as a motivational, musical audio guide you can use during your walks, are available by calling (800) 207-8633, or online at www.arthritis.org. The Arthritis Foundation now has an annual Arthritis Walk held at cities nationwide each April. Call (800) 283-7800 or search the Arthritis Foundation Web site to find your local chapter.

motion, reducing your chance of muscle strain and additional pain.

Swimming and water aerobics are highly recommended as a cardiovascular workout, because little stress is placed on your joints. As noted in Chapter Eight, the Arthritis Foundation offers an aquatic exercise program, AFAP (or AFYAP when offered at YMCAs), designed for those with chronic pain, and sells a do-it-yourself water-exercise video, *Pool Exercise Program,* as well.

Bicycling. Riding a stationary or standard bicycle can offer aerobic exercise without placing much stress on damaged or painful hips, knees or feet. Some stationary bicycles have movable handles that exercise your upper body as well, offering additional cardiovascular benefit.

When beginning a cycling routine, don't pedal faster than 5 to 10 miles per hour. As you become fitter, increase your speed and/or add resistance. If you have knee pain or osteoarthritis of the knee, consult your doctor or physical therapist to determine if bicycling is an acceptable exercise for you, as you may be at risk of injury. If you ride a standard bicycle, use proper safety equipment and choose a safe, well-paved route.

Dancing. Dance is a great cardiovascular exercise method that's rarely boring, because it's set to your favorite music. As old as civilization itself, dance is a part of every world culture. There are many different types of dance: disco, folk, square, step, country line, ballroom, ballet, tap, jazz. You can dance alone, with a partner or in a group.

To dance for fitness, all you really need is a little space, some comfortable clothes and quality shoes, and some music. There are

# Walking Progression For Fitness

The following suggested progressive walking routine should help you get your program started and build endurance and stamina. When you can walk for a total of 10 minutes at a time (including a warm-up and cool-down period), try this progression chart to gradually build your walking fitness program. If you can already walk for longer than 10 minutes at a time, enter the chart at your current level and progress from there.

| Week | Time Duration Per Walking Session* | Frequency Per Week |
|---|---|---|
| 1 | 10 minutes | 3-5 times |
| 2 | 15 minutes | 3-5 times |
| 3 | 20 minutes | 3-5 times |
| 4 | 25 minutes | 3-5 times |
| 5 | 30 minutes | 3-5 times |
| 6 | 30-35 minutes | 3-5 times |
| 7 | 30-40 minutes | 3-5 times |
| 8 | 30-45 minutes | 3-5 times |
| 9 | 30-50 minutes | 3-5 times |

10 and onward: Keep your walks at 30-60 minutes per session, 3-5 times per week. Gradually increase your intensity until you are in the moderate range (if you are not doing so yet).

* Includes warm up and cool down, but not stretching.

dance classes in every community, where instructors can teach you how to perform particular dance steps and monitor your progress. Dance classes can also be social, and having a set time when you dance with your friends can encourage you to keep it up. If you do wish to join a dance class, talk to the instructor beforehand about your chronic pain or health condition. You need to find a class that is suitable for your needs. Ask the instructor about what type of clothing or footwear you need to have to participate safely.

If you would rather not dance in a formal class setting, all you have to do is turn on some tunes and get moving! Your living room will do just fine for a dance floor. Or, try stepping out to a local dance club with your spouse, family or friends.

Use good judgment when dancing for fitness. Don't try to push yourself to dance more vigorously, or to copy difficult steps, before you know you are ready. Wear comfortable clothing that allows you to move freely and perspire. Dancing should be a fun way to work up a sweat.

# Head-to-Toe Water Workout

Try these exercises at your community pool, in your hot tub or as part of an aquatic class.

### 1) Knee Lift

Step 1: Stand with your left side against the pool wall.

Step 2: Bend your right knee and bring your thigh parallel to the water's surface, or as high as you can. (Cup your hands behind your knee for extra support.)

Step 3: Straighten your knee, lower your leg. Repeat on the left side.

### 2) Arm Circles

Step 1: Raise both arms forward a few inches below water level. (Keep elbows straight.)

Step 2: Make small circles (softball size) with your arms. Increase the circles to basketball size, then decrease.

Step 3: Alternate between inward and outward circles. (Don't raise your arms out of the water or let them cross.)

### 3) Side Bend

Step 1: Place your feet shoulder-width apart and relax your knees.

Step 2: Bend slowly toward the right. Return to starting position and bend to the left. (Don't bend forward or twist or turn your trunk.)

Step 3: You can try the exercise with your arms hanging at your sides, with your hand sliding down your thigh as you bend. Repeat on your left side.

### 4) Ankle Bend

Step 1: Place your hands on your hips or hold the side of the pool for support.

Step 2: Bend your foot up, then down.

Step 3: Repeat with your other foot.

## Alternative Exercise Methods

Some people find exercise boring or unpleasant. Gentle, alternative forms of exercise can seem easier and more interesting for some people. For people with chronic pain, a gentler form of exercise that still has endorphin-boosting, flexibility-increasing and aerobic benefits can seem like the best option.

It's likely that one of the following forms of exercise is taught in your area. Get instruction from a qualified professional so you perform the exercises properly, get the most benefit from them, and reduce your chances of injury or strain.

Yoga. Practiced by an increasing number of Americans in recent years, *yoga* has been a staple exercise routine for millions of people in India for centuries. Yoga is part of the traditional Indian healing philosophy known as *Ayurveda*.

There are many types of yoga. Some forms are gentle and others are more energetic or strenuous, causing you to break into a sweat. Hatha yoga is the gentle, most common kind of yoga, and it involves gentle stretching movements and balancing exercises known as postures that condition the whole body.

Practicing yoga regularly (you can do it daily) improves flexibility, balance and strength, because it involves stretching as well as bearing the weight of your body. Yoga is also relaxing and often includes meditation or deep breathing. Yoga is taught at many special centers, exercise clubs or spas, as well as through instructional tapes and videos. If you have chronic pain, learn yoga from a trained professional before trying routines on your own.

Tai chi. In China, where *tai chi* began, this combination of graceful motions is considered a martial art, like karate or tae kwon do. But tai chi doesn't look like fighting. Tai chi's controlled movements require grace and precision. Luckily, almost anyone can learn the simple, gentle movements of tai chi, gaining its health benefits.

Research studies show tai chi improves balance, reducing the risk of dangerous falls and injuries. Tai chi is increasingly popular among people with back pain or arthritis. Explore videotapes that instruct you in the practice of tai chi, books about tai chi, or local tai chi classes at community centers and health clubs. Check your local chapter of the Arthritis Foundation to see if there are tai chi for arthritis classes in your area.

Qi Gong. *Qi gong* (pronounced *chee kung*) is another ancient Asian practice that aims to promote health and the body's natural healing ability. As we learned in Chapter Seven, qi is the Chinese term for the natural energy flow and balance in the body.

There are several forms of qi gong, which involve meditation, breathing exercises and movements. Qi gong exercises seem less graceful than tai chi moves, and, like yoga, there are some more vigorous styles of qi gong. But qi gong exercises are appropriate for people of all ages and abilities, and can even be done from a bed or wheelchair.

Few studies show qi gong's benefits for pain relief, but one 1998 study of people with fibromyalgia who used qi gong along with meditation practices reported improvement in depression, pain and ability to function. Qi gong is taught at many community centers or health clubs nationwide.

Pilates. The *Pilates* method of exercise started in the 1920s, and it's becoming increasingly popular throughout the U.S. Pilates conditions and strengthens the body through specific exercises that emphasize proper body alignment, injury prevention and breathing.

While other exercises may focus on various parts of the body or on the body as a whole, Pilates really concentrates on the role of the back and spine in overall health. Pilates exercises may be difficult to perform at first, which is why it's essential to receive proper instruction and supervision in this technique. Pilates involves strengthening and stretching exercises to develop the muscles in the lower back and abdomen so they can provide firm support for your whole body's movements. Pilates aims to promote proper spinal alignment and stabilization. Usually taught in special Pilates centers, classes at health clubs or at physical therapy clinics, you perform the exercises on a special bench-like piece of equipment.

As we have learned, managing your chronic pain isn't simple – it requires a comprehensive approach from you and your doctor. Managing your pain can require making positive changes to your lifestyle, including improving your diet, quitting bad habits like smoking, taking your medications as prescribed and getting proper rest and exercise. One factor that may increase your pain, even if you do all of those healthful things, is stress. In the next chapter, we will look at how stress may play a role in chronic pain, and offer strategies for keeping stress at bay.

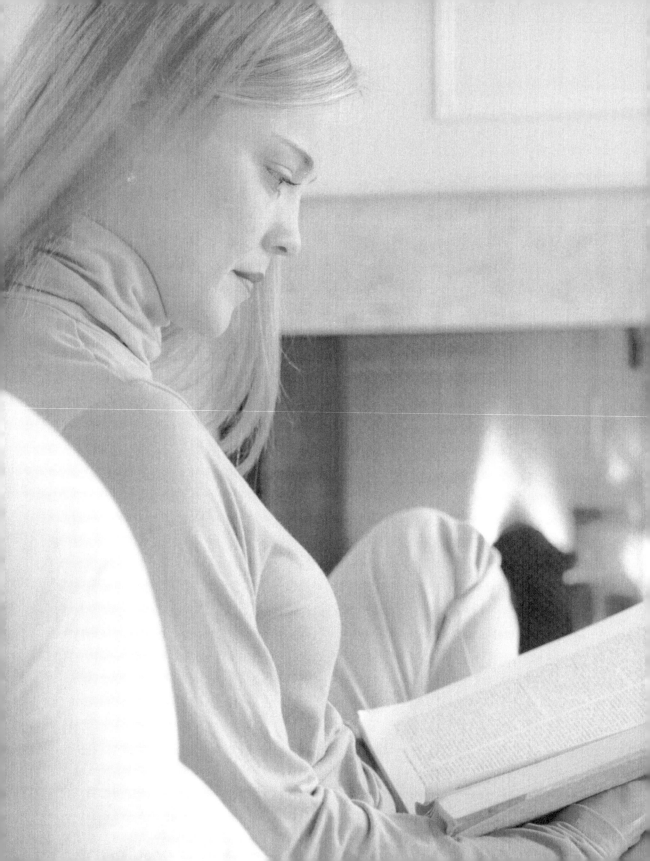

# Reducing
# Painful Stress

10

# CHAPTER 10: REDUCING PAINFUL STRESS

It's a proven fact: Stress can make pain worse. Stress may also cause pain in some cases.

How does this happen? When you are "stressed out," your muscles tense, causing pain. Your heart rate and body temperature increase. In reaction to stress, your body secretes the hormone *adrenaline*. Adrenaline, which comes from the adrenal glands near the kidneys, is your body's natural response mechanism to a frightening or dangerous situation. But when you have constant or regular stress, your body continues to pump adrenaline. It never shuts off, and your body cannot recover from a heightened emergency state. This stressed-out state is exhausting.

For someone with chronic pain due to arthritis, fibromyalgia, back pain, nerve damage or other diseases, this constant state of stress can be dangerous. This state of emergency puts too much strain on your heart, lungs and other organs. When you are in constant stress, adding to your chronic pain, you may seek out alcohol, cigarettes or drugs, abusing these substances in an unhealthy, dangerous way.

So controlling stress is vital for someone in chronic pain. Learning to relax – something that seems simple but actually requires concentration and effort – could save your life.

## WHAT IS STRESS?

Stress has become one of the most common buzzwords of our time. Almost everyone mentions stress on a daily basis: "I'm so stressed out at work from the pressure to make higher sales." "I'm having so much stress because my mother-in-law is coming to town for a visit." "The bills keep piling up and it's causing me to feel stress." Stress is something you feel all over, both in your mind and your body.

A person with chronic pain is highly susceptible to stress and its effects. Chronic pain never lets up, so the person in pain may feel overwhelmed by their condition and feel hopeless. Family members and friends may grow impatient or intolerant of the person's condition and not offer the support necessary, leading to stress. It may be more difficult for a person with chronic pain to keep up with their job requirements or goals, leading to even more stress.

Stress is defined as mental or physical tension, and it affects a person both mentally and physically in many cases. Stress causes mental reactions like anxiety, worry, fear, anger and nervousness. When stressed, you might snap at someone without meaning to act that way. Stress can also cause strong physical reactions, such as stomach upset, headaches, muscle tension or pain, perspiration, heart palpitations, tightened jaw and teeth grinding. Stress can lead you to engage in unhealthy practices, such as overeating, smoking, drinking alcohol or abusing drugs. So stress is a serious health threat, and needs to be addressed as such.

Stress may be caused by mental anxiety, tension or pressure, but the reactions can be physical in nature. When we face stress from any source, our bodies respond by releasing hormones like adrenaline and cortisol into the bloodstream. These hormones increase your heart rate, blood pressure and tense muscles. Why? This physical reaction probably stems from the earliest stages of human evolution, when humans faced life-or-death dangers on a regular basis. To respond to dangerous situations, they developed a physical emergency response system: The hormones released would put their whole bodies on alert status, something now called the "fight or flight response." In this state, we are intensely aware of the danger and ready to fight with all our might or run like crazy to survive.

This kind of response works most of the time. The stress response is beneficial during real emergencies or high-pressure situations. When the stressful situation is over, the body's vital signs should return to normal levels. Sometimes, as in the case with many people in chronic pain, they do not.

Stress levels in our modern society often remain high for sustained periods of time. You may experience stress daily from your job, traffic, your family or your health problems. If you can't release the tension after a stressful situation (such as being stuck in traffic), your body may begin to respond to every slightly stressful situation as if it's an emergency. This constant stress can wear down on every part of your body and mind. Just as it's bad for your car to "race the engine" constantly, it's bad for your body to race without a break.

People in chronic pain don't get a break from their pain and other symptoms. They may not sleep well, so they can't recharge their energy stores. Day after day, it becomes more difficult to deal with life in a positive, healthy way. You may find yourself reaching overload and notice the results. You could become more accident-prone. You might make more mistakes than usual. You might not sleep well and find it impossible to get a good night's sleep. These are signs that you need to try to relieve some of the stress in your life. Without releasing the tension and getting good sleep, your pain may worsen.

## Easing Stress Step by Step

Relaxation needs to occur one step at a time. You may have to learn methods of relaxation that work for you. Understandably, you may encounter problems that make it impossible to avoid stress. Nobody can avoid stress completely. When you have health problems, you can find even ordinary challenges very stressful. You may find it difficult to calm down after you have resolved the challenge. You might find yourself getting angry with family members, friends, coworkers, your doctor or even your pain itself.

But learning and practicing techniques for relaxation can help you manage stressful episodes in a healthier way. This chapter contains some proven techniques for healthy relaxation. You will have to practice them on your own, and find what works for you. Your doctor may be able to suggest methods to help you fight stress. If necessary, he can prescribe medications, like tranquilizers, antidepressants, anti-anxiety drugs or sedatives, to help you control stress or sleep better. Some alternative treatments can help reduce stress too.

The first step in controlling stress is to recognize the causes of stress. This is called identifying stressors. Stressors are the actual triggers to your stress. They can be anything, even supposedly joyful or simple things: visits from relatives for the holidays, leading a meeting at work, going to the doctor, meeting your daughter's new fiancé for the first time, packing for a trip, taking your car for a repair. Often, the stressor is not something you pinpoint right away. You may tell yourself that you don't mind certain tasks or activities, when in fact you do find the situation or activity stressful. For example, you may love going on a vacation with your family. But when you think about it, going to the airport – parking the car, going through ticketing and security, getting on the plane – are stressful. So these aspects of travel cause you to become tense.

The second step is recognizing how you respond to stress. These are the reactions to the stressor. Since stressors may not always be obvious to you, linking your physical or emotional reactions may be difficult also. For example, you may have headaches on occasion. Are these headaches caused by a stressor? Write down when you have headaches so that you can note patterns. Do you get one every time you face a stressful situation? If so, stress may be causing the headaches, not your drugs or your allergies. Keeping a journal may help you identify what causes your stress and how you respond to it.

After you identify what causes your stress and how you respond to stress, the third step is to develop coping strategies, so you deal with stress more effectively and avoid or reduce your reactions. There are many unhealthy strategies for coping with stress: smoking, drinking, abusing drugs, yelling, fighting, self-blame, avoidance. These strategies may be easy ways to "deal" with stress in your life, but they will only increase your tension, damage your relationships and, eventually, worsen your pain.

Find coping strategies that are positive, healthy and effective. This chapter contains some suggested coping strategies to help you. You may have to experiment to find the one that works for you.

## Stress Journal

You might be able to eliminate stress by learning what causes it and how you respond to it, both physically and emotionally. Physical reactions might include headaches, stomachaches, muscle tension or breaking out into a sweat. Emotional reactions might include anxiety, panicking, getting angry or crying.

By keeping a daily stress journal for a week or two, you'll discover patterns in your stress and the reactions or symptoms of stress. Once you know what causes your stress and how you react to it, you will know when you need to apply the stress-reduction methods discussed in this chapter.

Try keeping your own stress journal (see sample above). Write down not only what situations cause your stress, but how you felt before, during and after the situation. Does your chronic

# Sample Stress Journal

| Date | Time | Cause of Stress | Physical Symptoms | Emotional Symptoms |
|------|------|-----------------|-------------------|--------------------|
| 4/18 | 7 a.m. | Cooking breakfast for children | Fast heartbeat, tightening back muscles | Feel rushed |
| 4/18 | 8 a.m. | Stuck in traffic | Headache, heart beating | Screamed at other cars |
| 4/23 | 1 p.m. | Presentation for boss | Fast heartbeat, dry throat, back pain afterward | Anxious, nervous |

pain make you feel worried about your job performance? Do you feel that your family and friends don't understand your pain, so you become anxious before social outings? Do you become uncontrollably angry in traffic, honking your horn continuously? Does your heart beat faster? All of these facts, when you write them in your journal, will begin to show patterns in your feelings and behaviors. You may wish to share this journal with your doctor or therapist and discuss what responses you can try.

## Learning To Relax

Relaxation therapies can be done almost anywhere and at any time. Some may be more appropriate for times when you are at home and have more time to truly relax. Relaxation is not just kicking off your shoes with a beer and the TV remote control. Relaxation is a more organized, strategic activity designed to bring your body processes like heartbeat and temperature back to normal. You will learn to relax your muscles and reduce excess pain.

Here, we will share a few successful stress-management techniques. Try them and see what works for you.

Deep Breathing. To practice deep breathing, sit in a comfortable chair with your feet on the floor and your arms at your sides. Close your eyes and breathe in deeply, saying to yourself , "I am….," then slowly breathe out, while saying, "…relaxed."

Continue to breathe slowly, silently repeating something to yourself such as, "My hands …are warm; my feet …are warm; my breathing …is deep and smooth; my heartbeat …is calm and steady; I feel calm …and at peace."

Always coordinate the words you speak with your breathing.

Distraction techniques. Distraction techniques, like the physical retraining methods discussed in Chapter Eight, aim to teach your mind to focus on something other than your stress. Your mind kicks into a subconscious response pattern when you experience a stressful episode. This pattern includes physical and emotional reactions to stress and pain. But you can learn to control your mind so this response mechanism is interrupted. This does not mean that you will ignore the stress, only that you can learn to put it in perspective.

By reading your stress journal, identify common causes of your stress: morning commute traffic, doctor's appointments, parent/teacher conferences, phone conversations with your mother-in-law. You know these things cause stress and you know how you typically react. So anticipate the stress and how you will handle it. Create a strategy for what you will do once the stressful situation is over – such as going to the mall, taking a hot bath or going for a walk with your dog. Or, try imagining something really pleasant during the stressful episode. Perhaps you can think about happy times spent with your kids, or dream vacations you would love to take, or your favorite football team winning the Super Bowl. You may feel, at the time, as if the problem will last forever. It won't! By thinking of the enjoyable and relaxing things you will do afterward, you can distract your mind from the stress.

Guided Imagery. Guided imagery techniques also distract you from your stress. They are highly focused fantasies. You can do them anywhere – on the bus, at home or in your doctor's waiting room.

To practice guided imagery, close your eyes, take a deep breath and hold it for several seconds. Breathe out gradually, feeling your body relax as you breathe.

Think about a place you have been where you felt safe, pain-free and comfortable. Imagine it in as much detail as possible. Fantasize the sounds – waves crashing against the sand, seagulls calling overhead, the wind blowing. Think of smells, tastes and sights – saltwater breezes, cooking hotdogs, soft sand between your toes, coconut-scented lotion, the warm sun on your face.

Try to recapture and retain the positive feelings you had in this pleasant place and time. Remember them and keep them in your mind. Use this image to help you through painful or stressful times. Take several deep breaths and enjoy feeling calm and peaceful for a few minutes. Open your eyes.

Progressive relaxation. Progressive relaxation is a therapy in which the body's muscles, from head to toe, are progressively tensed and then relaxed. Progressive relaxation is a popular form of stress management, and it can also help you relax tight, tense muscles that make pain worse. Progressive relaxation is very useful for people in chronic pain. You may wish to do some basic flexibility or stretching exercises first so your muscles and tissues are properly limber.

Close your eyes and take a deep breath, filling your chest and breathing all the way down to your abdomen.

Breathe out, letting your stress flow out with the air.

Start with your feet and calves. Slowly flex and tighten your muscles. Hold for several seconds, then release the flex and relax your muscles. Gradually work your way through your major muscle groups using the same technique: upper legs, buttocks, stomach and torso, upper arms, lower arms and fingers, shoulders and neck, then to your jaw and face.

Continue breathing deeply and enjoy the feeling of relaxation before opening your eyes.

Visualization. Visualization is a technique that is very similar to distraction and guided imagery. When you have chronic pain, you often feel out of control. Pain and disease seem to control your life instead. Visualization techniques help reduce your stress and pain by allowing you to imagine yourself in control. You visualize yourself as the one in charge, and imagine yourself doing the things you love to do but often feel you cannot do. For example, visualize climbing a mountain or winning a marathon. By focusing on doing the things you want to do and enjoy doing, you are not focusing on the things that cause you stress.

Visualization exercise 1: Concentrate on something pleasant from your past, like the beach scene discussed before. Or imagine a new and better situation. It's creative fantasizing: Imagine yourself as a movie star accepting an award or making the big, lucrative deal at work.

Visualization exercise 2: Concentrate on symbols that represent your pain or stress in different parts of your body. Imagine that

painful back muscles are bright red. Then, visualize them as turning gradually into cool, soothing blue.

Visualization exercise 3: Concentrate on an image of your pain as a little green monster. Lock the monster in a metal garbage can. Shut the lid, lock it and put it in a dumpster to be hauled away.

## Sample Relaxation Exercises

Here are some other useful relaxation exercises to help you control stress and pain. First, find a comfortable, safe, quiet place to perform the exercise. Focus on your breathing. Concentrate on fresh breaths coming in and tension breathing out.

Then try one or more of these exercises. If you find one that really works for you, do it any time you feel stressed or in pain.

Pain Drain: Feel within your body and note where you experience pain or tension. Imagine that the pain or tension is turning into a liquid substance. This heavy liquid flows down through your body and through your fingers and toes. Allow the pain to drain from your body in a steady flow. Now, imagine that a gentle stream flows down over your head . . . and further dissolves the pain . . . into a liquid that continues to drain away. Enjoy the sense of comfort and well-being that follows.

Disappearing Pain: Notice any tension or pain that you are experiencing. Imagine that the pain takes the form of an object, or of several objects. It can be fruit, pebbles, crystals or anything else that comes to mind. Pick up each piece of pain, one at a time, and place it in a magic box.

As you drop each piece into the box, it dissolves into nothingness. Now, again survey your body to see if any pieces remain, and remove them. Imagine that your body is lighter now, and allow yourself to experience a feeling of comfort and well-being. Enjoy this feeling of tranquility and repose.

Healing Potion: Imagine you are in a drugstore that is stocked with bottles and jars of exotic potions. Each potion has a special magical quality. Some are of pure white light, others are lotions, balms and creams, and yet others contain healing vibrations. As you survey the many potions, choose one that appeals to you. It may even have your name on the container.

Open the container and cover your body with that magical potion. As you apply it, let any pain or tension slowly melt away, leaving you with a feeling of comfort and well-being. Imagine that you place the container in a special spot and that it continually renews its contents for future use.

## Writing Your Stress Away

Many people use a diary to record their feelings or thoughts about their life. The practice of writing down your fears, hopes, dreams and beliefs can be fun, but it can also help you control stress. How? When you write out your feelings, you can put things in perspective, identify problems and solutions, and see patterns in your behavior and in your life that you can change for the better.

Research supports the idea that writing in a diary can help you cope with the stress and pain of chronic illness. One study of people with rheumatoid arthritis showed that those who regularly wrote about their most stressful life events experienced a 28 percent reduction in overall disease symptoms.

Stress can contribute to disease activity. This study also shows that reducing stress – specifically by writing about emotionally troubling events or issues – may decrease the severity of your disease. Here are some tips for starting your own diary.

- **Choose pen and paper – or a screen.** Find a bound diary with a pretty cover, a handy spiral notebook, or a blank tablet with lots of open space to write in. Or, if you prefer a computer, start a private file of documents and add pictures or choose particular fonts and colors that suit you. The Arthritis Foundation publishes a blank book specifically designed for people with arthritis. *Toward Healthy Living: A Wellness Journal* is a spiral-bound, glossy diary with inspiring quotes in the borders of pages, as well as charts to track daily changes in pain and mood. To order, call (800) 207-8633 or log on to www.arthritis.org.
- **Don't worry about grammar or spelling.** Your diary is for your eyes only. Make sure family members know that this journal is not to be read by them. You don't need to impress anyone with handwriting, proper grammar or spelling. Use a thesaurus or dictionary if you find it helpful, but don't

worry about expressing your thoughts in any other way except how you normally do.

- **Choose a relaxing time and place to write regularly.** Don't try to write in your diary while you're cooking dinner for the family. Pick a time and place with few distractions so you can write without being interrupted. This time is for you alone.
- **Let it flow.** Express your emotions freely. No one else will have to see what you write, and you need to feel comfortable expressing your emotions no matter what they are.
- **Get help if you need it.** Writing in your diary may stir painful feelings. If you find these emotions difficult to deal with, consider turning to someone who can help. Your pain and stress may be too much for you to handle alone. Your doctor can refer you to a psychologist or licensed therapist, or you can consult a counselor, minister, rabbi or other trained clergyman. Take your diary to counseling sessions if you like, and share certain feelings you would like to discuss.

Stress doesn't have to take over your life. It's hard enough to handle daily life and responsibilities with chronic pain. You have a lot to juggle – medications, doctor's visits, family and friends, job, bills and pain. Constant stress will only make things worse, and could even seriously hurt you physically and emotionally. Avoid tense situations or aggravating people if you can. Try these techniques to learn to relax, or get help if you need it. Stress can be managed just as pain can be managed: With your effort and with help from those around you.

# CONCLUSION

Chronic pain is a serious and growing problem in our society. Despite advances in medicine and understanding of the human body, more and more people are in poor general health and experiencing pain. Thankfully, there is hope.

There are new, powerful medications designed to attack the causes of disease and pain. There are useful, natural strategies to help people reduce their own pain and relax during stressful times. There is new research on how to eat right, lose weight and exercise to achieve the maximum state of fitness no matter how old you are. There are organizations that offer helpful resources for people in chronic pain, resources that include health information, exercise courses, lifestyle management classes, support groups, social outings and 24-hour Web sites where you can talk to others in chronic pain and experts with answers to medical questions. The Internet has made a wealth of health and pain-management information available to almost everyone, everywhere, at any time.

The Arthritis Foundation, which published this book, is devoted to the cause of fighting pain. The mission of the Arthritis Foundation is to improve lives through leadership in the prevention, control and cure of arthritis and related diseases. The organization raises much-needed funds for medical research and conducts educational programs for people nationwide.

Reach out in your own community and find helpful resources and guidance for living with pain. Ask your doctor for advice or strategies to help manage your pain. Learn more about the cause of your pain and what new medical advances may help you treat your pain more effectively. If you find new research and want to know more, ask your doctor. Contact drug manufacturers to learn more about their latest pain-management medications or treatments. Read up on studies about alternative treatments or new drugs to see what works and what may be a waste of time.

Educating yourself, dedicating yourself to good health habits and maintaining an open dialogue with your health-care professionals are three key steps to managing your pain. While it would be great if a magic pill could erase your pain, in most cases, that won't happen. But there are many things you can do to manage your pain and live a fuller, more active life. Pain doesn't have to win this battle – with the strategies in this book and others on the horizon, it's our hope that you will win and have a happy, less painful life.

## RESOURCES FOR GOOD LIVING

The Arthritis Foundation, the only national, voluntary health organization that works for the more than 70 million Americans with arthritis or related diseases, offers many valuable resources through more than 150 offices nationwide. The chapter that serves your area has information, products, classes and other services to help you take control of your arthritis or related condition. To find the chapter nearest you, call (800) 283-7800 or search the Arthritis Foundation Web site at www.arthritis.org.

## Programs and Services

- **Physician referral:** Most Arthritis Foundation chapters can provide a list of doctors in your area who specialize in the evaluation and treatment of arthritis and arthritis-related diseases.
- **Exercise programs:** The Arthritis Foundation sponsors, develops and coordinates exercise programs for people with arthritis, featuring specially-trained instructors. They include:
- **Walk With Ease:** This course allows participants to develop a walking plan that meets their individual needs, accompanied by the Arthritis Foundation book *Walk With Ease: Your Guide to Walking for Better Health, Improved Fitness and Less Pain.* A new audio walking guide is now available to use during your walking routines, with guidelines, upbeat music and inspiring motivation. In addition, a *Walk With Ease* group leader's manual is available to help you start and lead a walking group in your area.
- **PACE** (People with Arthritis Can Exercise): These courses feature gentle movements to increase joint flexibility, range of motion, stamina and muscle strength. Accompanying videos at different fitness levels are available for home use.

- **Arthritis Foundation Aquatic Program:** These water exercise programs help relieve strain on muscles and joints. An accompanying PEP (Pool Exercise Program) video is available for home use. When taught at participating YMCA centers, this program is known as AFYAP (Arthritis Foundation YMCA Aquatics Program).
- **Self-Help Courses:** The Arthritis Foundation sponsors mutual-support groups — the Fibromyalgia Self-Help Course and the Arthritis Self-Help Course — that provide opportunities for discussion and problem solving with peers. In addition, these Arthritis Foundation courses help people actively manage their particular disease through exercise, medications, relaxation techniques, pain management, nutrition and more.

## Information and Products

Find the latest information about arthritis, including research, medications, government advocacy, programs and services through one of the many information resources offered by the Arthritis Foundation:

- **www.arthritis.org:** Information about arthritis is available 24 hours a day on the Internet at the Arthritis Foundation's interactive, comprehensive Web site. Find news about arthritis, ways to get involved, and a variety of useful arthritis products, including books, brochures, videos and more. In addition, the Arthritis Foundation has a new interactive self-management guide for people with arthritis, *Connect and Control: Your Online*

*Arthritis Action Guide.* Via questionnaire responses, *Connect and Control* helps participants create a customized management program for their unique situation.

- **Arthritis Answers:** Call toll-free at (800) 283-7800 for 24-hour, automated information about arthritis and Arthritis Foundation resources. Trained volunteers and staff are also available at your local Arthritis Foundation chapter to answer questions or refer you to physicians and other resources. For general questions about arthritis, you can also call (404) 872-7100 ext. 1, or email questions to help@arthritis.org.

- **Publications:** The Arthritis Foundation offers many publications to educate people with arthritis, as well as their families and friends, about diagnosis, medications, exercise, diet, pain management and more.

- **Books:** The Arthritis Foundation publishes a variety of books on arthritis to help you learn to understand and manage your condition, live a healthier life, and cope with the emotional challenges that come with a chronic illness. Order books directly at www.arthritis.org or by calling (800) 207-8633. All Arthritis Foundation books are available at your local bookstore or through online booksellers.

- **Brochures:** The Arthritis Foundation offers brochures containing concise, understand- able information on the many arthritis-related diseases and conditions. Topics include surgery, the latest medications, guidance for working with your doctors and self-managing your illness. Single copies are available free of charge at www.arthritis.org or by calling (800) 283-7800.

- ***Arthritis Today:*** This award-winning bimonthly magazine provides the latest information on research, new treatments, trends and tips from experts and readers to help you manage arthritis. A one-year subscription to *Arthritis Today* is included when you become a member of the Arthritis Foundation. Annual membership is $20 and helps fund research to find cures for arthritis. Call (800) 933-0032 for information.

- ***Kids Get Arthritis, Too:*** This newsletter focusing on juvenile rheumatic diseases, is published six times a year. Features speak to children and teens with the illness as well as to their parents. Stories examine the latest news in diagnosis, treatment and research of children's rheumatic diseases, as well as helpful ways kids can cope with their illnesses and the challenges they bring. This newsletter is now a benefit of membership in the Arthritis Foundation for people affected by juvenile rheumatic diseases. For information, call (800) 283-7800.

# Glossary & Index

## Pain Management

# Glossary

## A

**ACETAMINOPHEN** – The most commonly used analgesic medicine. The active ingredient in the brand-name pain-reliever *Tylenol*.

**ACID REFLUX** – Painful condition marked by stomach acid flowing back up into the esophagus, leading to heartburn and gastrointestinal damage.

**ACTIVE INGREDIENT** – The element in a medication or supplement that performs the treatment function in the body, as opposed to inactive ingredients, which are fillers to give the product taste, shape or binding.

**ACUTE** – Lasting for a short or contained period of time, as opposed to pain or illness that is chronic, or long-lasting and possibly permanent.

**ACUPUNCTURE** – Medicine technique created in ancient China in which thin needles are used to puncture the body at specific sites along energy pathways call meridians. Widely considered an alternative therapy, but gaining acceptance in Western medicine for pain relief. *Acupressure* is another form of this treatment, but one involving hand pressure rather than needle punctures.

**ADDICTION** – Dangerous reliance on and use of a drug or other treatment. May be of a physical or psychological nature.

**ADRENALINE** – Hormone produced by the adrenal glands near the kidneys. Adrenaline is produced during times of emotional or physical excitement.

**ALEXANDER TECHNIQUE** – Exercise-related movement therapy aimed at teaching the body less painful ways to move.

**ANALGESIC** – A medication used to treat pain, including acetaminophen and narcotic drugs. *Topical analgesics,* or rub-on ointments that temporarily treat pain, are also included in this category.

**ANEMIA** – A state of having less than the normal amount of red blood cells. May be a symptom of various problems.

**ANESTHESIA** – Chemicals that induce a partial or complete loss of sensation. Used for temporary pain relief, or to reduce sensation for surgery and other medical procedures.

**ANESTHESIOLOGIST** – Physician specializing in administering anesthesia during surgical procedures or other medical treatment. This specialty also includes the field of *pain medicine*, the comprehensive treatment of pain. Some anesthesiologists are also pain medicine specialists who consult patients on how to treat pain.

**ANKYLOSING SPONDYLITIS (AS)** – A form of arthritis that mainly affects the spine and sacroiliac joints (at the base of the spine where it attaches to the pelvis). In severe cases, people with AS may develop a fused and rigid spine.

**ANTICONVULSANTS** – Medicines designed to suppress convulsions.

**ANTIBODIES** – Cells that help the body's immune system fight against foreign agents that may cause disease.

**ANTIPYRETIC** – Medicines designed to lower elevated body temperature or fever.

**ANTISPASTICS** – Medicines designed to suppress spasms or seizures. Also called antispasmodic.

**AROMATHERAPY** – Alternative therapy involving the inhaling or application of particular scented substances (such as oils) in order to relieve pain, reduce inflammation or promote relaxation.

**ARTHRODESIS** – a surgical procedure in which the two bones that form a joint are prepared and held in place allowing them to fuse into a single, immovable unit

**ARTHROPLASTY** – Also called joint replacement surgery, a procedure in which a damaged joint is surgically removed and replaced with a synthetic one

**ARTHROSCOPY** – Surgical procedure in which a thin, lighted scope is inserted into the joint through a small incision, allowing the joint's interior to be viewed on a monitor.

**ARTHROSCOPE** – Instrument used in arthroscopy to view the inside of the joint during surgery.

**ASPIRATION** – The process of removing fluid or cells from the body through a needle, often used in removing fluid from joints in a variety of diagnostic tests and treatment procedures.

**ATROPHY** – A decrease in muscle mass due to extended lack of use or immobility.

**AUTOANTIBODIES** – Antibodies gone awry that attack the body's own cells instead of foreign cells that may cause disease.

# Glossary

**AUTOIMMUNE DISEASE** – A disease in which the immune system, which is designed to protect the body from foreign invaders such as viruses and bacteria, instead turns against and causes damage to the body's healthy tissue.

**AUTONOMIC NERVES** – Nerves that regulate normal body functions, such as heart rate, breathing, sweating, blood pressure and food digestion.

**AYURVEDA** – Healing tradition created in ancient India and incorporating various healing philosophies and techniques.

**BALNEOTHERAPY** – Therapeutic application of warm, mineral rich mud through application of packs or soaking in baths.

## B

**BENIGN** – A term for a tumor or mass that is no threat to the body and noncancerous. Usually benign masses are removed.

**BIOFEEDBACK** – The use of electronic instruments to measure body functions and feed that information back to you, allowing you to learn how to control body processes, such as heart rate or blood pressure, that are generally thought to be out of conscious control.

**BIOLOGIC RESPONSE MODIFIERS** – Agents derived from living sources, as opposed to synthesized chemicals, that target specific immune-system chemicals that play a role in the inflammation and damage of a disease while other leaving other immune-system components intact.

**BIOPSY** – A test performed on a piece of bodily tissue that is removed surgically, most often through a small incision. Depending on the piece of tissue examined, your doctor may use a biopsy to diagnose diseases of the joint, muscle, skin or blood vessels.

**BISPHOSPHONATES** — a class of medications that inhibit bone resorption and are used to treat bone diseases such as osteoporosis

**BONE SPUR** – A protruding outgrowth of bone, commonly on the heel, caused by disease or injury.

**BRACE** – A medical device used to hold a joint in place for proper movement, offering additional support for weak joints or muscles. Braces can be a temporary aid for reducing some pain.

**BURSA** – Small, fluid-filled sac that cushions and lubricates joints. Plural is bursae.

**BURSITIS** – Inflammation of the bursa.

## C

**CAPSAICIN** – Substance derived from the oil of hot cayenne peppers and used as a topical analgesic.

**CARPAL TUNNEL SYNDROME** – Painful neuropathic condition caused by a compression and irritation of the median nerve located in the wrist, often the result of repetitive overuse.

**CARTILAGE** — Smooth, rubbery tissue covering the ends of the bones at the joints, allowing the joint to move smoothly.

**CELL OXIDATION** – The natural process of cells breaking down over time due to oxidation, or exposure to oxygen, which is present throughout nature.

**CENTRAL NERVOUS SYSTEM** – The part of the body's nervous system that includes the brain and spinal cord, but not including the *peripheral nervous system*, or the network of nerves that spread throughout the body.

**CEREBRAL CORTEX** – The outer layer of gray matter on the brain.

**CHINESE MEDICINE** – Traditional Chinese healing philosophy and practices, including acupuncture, herbal treatments and qi gong.

**CHIROPRACTIC** – Practice of healing based on spinal manipulation and the belief that illness stems from misalignment of the spinal cord.

**CHIROPRACTOR** – A doctor of chiropractic (DC), who has four years of specialized training in chiropractic. Not a medical doctor.

**CHRONIC** – Lasting for a long time, usually defined as three months or more. Chronic pain and chronic conditions may also be permanent.

**COLLAGEN** – a protein that is the primary component of cartilage and other connective tissue

**COMPLEMENTARY THERAPY** – An alternative therapy that is used in conjunction with standard medical therapies, but not in place of these therapies. Can include healthy habits such as exercise, diet or relaxation techniques.

**COMPLEX REGIONAL PAIN SYNDROME** – See *reflex sympathetic dystrophy.*

# Glossary

COPAYMENT – A standard fee that a patient pays for a medical procedure or service.

CORTICOSTEROIDS — Hormones, including cortisol, naturally produced by the adrenal glands. Synthetic corticosteroids, can be produced and have powerful anti-inflammatory effects. They are sometimes called glucocorticoids or steroids.

COUNTERIRRITANTS – Topical analgesics that contain stimulating or cooling substances meant to provide a soothing counteraction to localized pain. Often contain oil of wintergreen, camphor, menthol or other substances that create a sensation of coolness.

COX-2 SPECIFIC INHIBITORS – A new class of NSAIDs, including celecoxib, rofecoxib and valdecoxib, that specifically inhibit COX-2, the prostaglandin related to inflammation.

CRANIAL MANIPULATION – Application of gentle pressure to the skull (cranium) in an attempt to relieve pain or tinnitus (chronic ringing in the ears). Usually performed by an osteopath or a chiropractor.

CRANIO-SACRAL THERAPY – Alternative therapy involving physical manipulation of the head, neck and spine. The philosophy behind Cranio-Sacral Therapy purports that pain results from an imbalance of fluids in these body parts.

CYTOKINES – Substances in the body's immune system that help fight disease. In autoimmune diseases, cytokines may go awry and destroy the body's components instead.

## D

DEGENERATIVE – Refers to diseases or conditions that worsen over time, deteriorating the body or its components in a gradual manner.

DEPENDENCE – A physical or emotional reliance for a drug that may be, in some cases, unhealthy. Differs from addiction, which connotes dangerous use of and need for a drug.

DERMATOMYOSITIS – See *polymyositis*.

DEXA – Short for dual-energy X-ray absorptiometry, a scan that measures bone density at the hip and spine to diagnose osteoporosis and evaluate bone density

DISABILITY – A state of being unable to perform basic functions. Also a legal term describing long-term, complete incapacity to work.

DMARDs – Short for disease-modifying antirheumatic drugs, a class of drugs that work to interfere with or alter the immune system's malfunctioning response in autoimmune diseases like rheumatoid arthritis.

DOSAGE – The amount of a drug's active ingredient that a person consumes in one measured allotment.

DOSE-PACK – Term for a contained supply of a medicine, such as corticosteroid, in which the dose of medicine is tapered gradually.

DURA MATER – The outer membrane covering the spinal cord. There is a risk of puncturing the dura mater in some pain injection procedures.

## E

EFFICACY – Effectiveness of a procedure or treatment.

ELECTROACUPUNCTURE – Acupuncture involving electronic stimulation in the needles used in the procedure.

ENDORPHINS – Hormones produced by the body in response to pain or heavy physical exertion, such as exercise.

ENKEPHALINS – Hormones similar to endorphins that may act as neurotransmitters.

EPICONDYLE – The area of the bone where the muscles are attached to the elbow.

EPIDURAL – Related to the space surrounding the dura, or fluid-filled sac around the spine. Anesthetic medicine may be injected into the epidural space to numb parts of the body during surgery or childbirth. Some chronic pain patients receive *epidural injections* as well.

EROSIONS – Areas where a structure is worn away or deteriorated. In the gastrointestinal system, refers to shallow, small ulcers that develop in the lining of the stomach or intestine, causing intense pain. Erosions can also occur in joints in osteoarthritis and other forms of arthritis.

ERYTHROCYTE SEDIMENTATION RATE (ESR) – Also referred to as *sed rate*, a test measuring how fast red blood cells (erythrocytes) clump together and fall to the bottom of a test tube like sediment.

# Glossary

## F

**FASCIA** – Fibrous tissues located beneath the skin. Fascia can become inflamed and painful. Some massage techniques involve manipulation of the fascia.

**FATIGUE** – A state of exhaustion usually marked by feelings of sleepiness, weariness or lack of energy. Fatigue may be a general sensation or confined to one organ, such as muscles.

**FELDENKRAIS METHOD** – Therapy involving exercises or physical techniques designed to train the person to move their body in a way that reduces pain and improves health.

**FIBROMYALGIA** – A syndrome characterized by widespread muscle pain, the presence of tender points (or points on the body that feel painful on pressure) and often debilitating fatigue and other symptoms.

**FIELD BLOCK INJECTIONS** – Another term for trigger point injections, or injections of corticosteroid directly into points of the body that may be triggers for painful reactions elsewhere in the body.

**FLARE** – An unusually severe episode of disease activity.

**FREE RADICAL** – A compound that is unstable and a possible contributor to cell degeneration. Free radicals are in the atmosphere as well as the body. Their role in cell metabolism, as well as the aging and disease process, is not fully understood at this time.

## G

**GATE CONTROL THEORY OF PAIN** – A common theory that holds that the flow of pain signals into the brain can be somehow reduced or manipulated, thereby lessening pain.

**GLUCOCORTICOIDS** – See corticosteroids.

**GOLFER'S ELBOW** – Similar to tennis elbow, but when the inside of the elbow is affected. The medical term is medial epicondylitis.

**GOUT** – a form of arthritis that occurs when uric acid builds up in the blood and deposits as crystals in the joints and other tissue. A joint affected by gout may be excruciatingly painful and shiny and purplish in appearance

**GUIDED IMAGERY** – Technique involving using concentrated focus on pleasant images as a distraction from pain.

## H

**HEALTH-CARE PROFESSIONAL** – Generally, any licensed professional consulting with a patient about health-care concerns.

**HELLERWORK** – Massage-based alternative practice incorporating methods to teach the person to move or hold their body in a less painful way.

**HEMATOMA** – A localized swelling or sac that is filled with blood.

**HERBAL SUPPLEMENTS** – Nutritional supplements that contain natural plant-derived substances and are meant to have therapeutic or health-promoting effects. Herbal supplement is a loosely applied term.

**HYALURONIC ACID** – a substance in the synovial fluid of the joints that give the fluid its viscosity and shock-absorbing properties.

**HYDROTHERAPY** – Therapeutic use of water pressure, such as in a whirlpool or spa bath, to relieve muscle or joint pain.

## I

**IDIOPATHIC PAIN** – Pain of unknown cause or origin.

**IN VITRO** – Literally "in glass," or in a test tube. A term describing a test performed in a test tube in a laboratory setting as opposed to being conducted in a clinical trial or on live creatures.

**IN VIVO** – Literally "in the living." A term describing something being done to live creatures, often referring to drug or supplement tests conducted in clinical trials on humans or animals.

**IMMUNE SYSTEM** – The body's system of organs and cells responsible for identifying and attacking foreign agents that may cause disease.

**IMPLANTABLE DEVICES** – Pain-relief devices that are surgically implanted inside a person's body. Some implantable devices are pumps that deliver steady doses of analgesic medicine, and others are electrical devices that deliver steady pulses of electrical stimulation.

**INFECTIOUS ARTHRITIS** – Form of arthritis that occurs when an infection settles in a joint or joints.

# Glossary

INFLAMMATION – Localized occurrence of swelling, warmth, redness and pain resulting from disease, infection, injury or irritation.

INITIAL CONSULTATION – The first time a patient meets with a health-care professional for examination.

INTEGRATIVE MEDICINE – Practice of incorporating alternative or natural medical techniques and therapies into a medical or allopathic philosophy of medicine.

INTERLEUKIN-1 – A protein produced by the body that contributes to inflammation in some cases.

INTERNIST – A medical doctor with additional years of training in internal medicine. Often, internists serve as primary-care physicians.

INTRACTABLE PAIN – Pain that cannot be effectively treated or that is not responding to any available pain treatment.

INTRAMUSCULAR INJECTION – Injection of a medicine or solution into muscle tissue.

INTRATHECAL – Related to the area around the spinal cord where pain receptor nerves are located. Anesthetic may be injected into the intrathecal space.

INTRAVENOUS – Into a vein. Some medicines are injected or infused by needle intravenously.

## J

JOINT – The juncture of two or more bones in the body. Some joints are rigid and others that allow the body to move in many different positions.

JOINT CAPSULE – The space where two bones meet in a joint, an area containing not only bone and cartilage but also nerves and soft tissues such as tendons, ligaments, muscles or bursae.

JUVENILE RHEUMATOID ARTHRITIS – a type of arthritis that occurs in children under age 16. There are three different forms of JRA, differentiated primarily by the number of joints they affect.

## K

KINESIOLOGY – The science or study of movement, particularly as applies to humans or other animals. Some chiropractors follow a philosophy of kinesiology and believe that some pain evolves from improper movement.

## L

LACTOSE INTOLERANCE – Inability to digest lactose, a component of milk and other dairy products, due to a deficiency of the lactase enzyme. A common condition marked by stomach upset and painful flatulence after ingestion of lactose.

LIGAMENTS – Bands of tough connective tissue that attach bones to bones and help keep them together at a joint.

LIMBIC CENTER – A part of the brain near the brainstem where pain signals may be processed.

LYME DISEASE – A form of infectious arthritis caused by the person acquiring the borrelia Burgdorferi bacterium, usually from the bite of an infected tick.

## M

MALIGNANT – Term for a tumor or mass that is cancerous, or growing and potentially harmful to the body.

MANIPULATION THERAPY – Alternative therapy involving the physical manipulation of a part of the body, such as the spine, neck or cranium.

MEDICAL DOCTOR – A licensed physician with a medical doctorate or MD degree. May be a specialist or general practice physician.

MEDICAL HISTORY – Record of a patient's personal health background, including diseases, injuries, surgical procedures, vaccinations, health habits or health problems the patient may have had, as well as family history of disease. May be formal or informal.

MEDITATION – Practice of using deep breathing and concentration exercises in order to promote relaxation.

MERIDIANS – In Chinese medicine, energy pathways throughout the body that an acupuncturist pricks to stimulate healthy energy flow or to reduce pain.

MESMERISM – Archaic term for hypnosis.

METHOTREXATE – One of the most common disease-modifying antirheumatic drugs, used for treating autoimmune diseases such as rheumatoid arthritis.

MOXIBUSTION – Form of acupuncture which also includes treatment with a burning cone of dried herb, such as mugwort.

# Glossary

MOTOR NERVES – Nerves that regulate the motion of your muscles, allowing you to move various body parts and other functions.

MRI — short for magnetic resonance imaging, MRI is a procedure in which a very strong magnet is used to pass a force through the body to create a clear, detailed image of a cross-section of the body

MUCUS – Thick, lubricating or coating fluid produced by many organs of the body.

MUSCLE – Soft tissues in the body that support other structures and act as a power source for all kinds of movement. There are different types of muscle, including skeletal muscle and the heart itself, also known as cardiac muscle.

## N

NARCOTIC – A drug derived from opium or opium-like materials that is used as a powerful analgesic, or pain reliever.

NATURAL MEDICINE – Alternative field of health care involving treating illness or pain through herbs, supplements and various non-medical methods.

NERVE BLOCK INJECTIONS – Injection treatments involving the numbing of nerve fibers that may be the source of chronic pain.

NERVE ENDINGS – Tiny endings of nerves that sense pain, temperature, texture or other stimuli. Includes the *nociceptors*, which perceive pain and other stimuli that might indicate harm to the body.

NERVOUS SYSTEM – The body's system of organs that collect and distribute data through a complex series of chemical and electrical signals, including nerves, the spinal cord and the brain.

NEUROHORMONES – Brain chemicals that play a role in the structure or function of the body's organs.

NEUROLOGIST – Medical doctor specializing in diseases or problems of the central nervous system.

NEUROPATHIC PAIN – Pain related to disease or malfunction of the nerves.

NEUROPLASTICITY – The theory that nerve cells and the pain process change in chronic pain.

NEUROSTIMULATORS – Devices surgically implanted in the body to deliver steady electrical pulses that treat nerve-related pain.

NEUROSURGEON – Neurologist with specialized training in surgical treatment of the central nervous system.

NEUROTRANSMITTERS – Body chemicals that help pain signals transmit and play a role in how the brain relays pain messages.

NOCICEPTORS – Peripheral nerve endings that sense pain.

NONSTEROIDAL ANTI-INFLAMMATORY DRUGS (NSAIDS) – A class of medications commonly used to ease the pain and inflammation of many forms of arthritis

NURSE – Health-care professional that assists doctors in many vital procedures and treating patients, as well as administering many basic health-care treatments on his or her own. Term may include registered nurses (RNs) and licensed practical nurses (LPNs).

NURSE PRACTITIONER – A registered nurse with additional training in a medical specialty. A nurse practitioner may be involved in either patient care or medical research.

## O

OBESE – A term describing a person who is more than 20 percent over their ideal body weight.

OCCUPATIONAL THERAPIST (OT) – A licensed health-care professional who is trained to evaluate the impact of disease or injury on daily activities, and advise patients on easier ways to perform activities or prescribe splints and assistive devices.

OCCUPATIONAL THERAPY – Health-care field focusing on the patient's ability to perform daily professional or personal tasks that may be impaired due to disease, surgery or injury, and training patients to find practical ways to do such tasks.

OPIATES – Also called opioids, drugs or substances derived from opium, which occurs naturally in the poppy plant.

ORTHOPAEDIC SURGEON – A doctor specializing in surgery involving the musculoskeletal system, including bones and joints.

OSTEOARTHRITIS (OA) – The most common form of arthritis, involving cartilage breakdown at certain joints resulting in pain and, in some cases, deformity.

# Glossary

**OSTEOPATHIC DOCTOR (DO)** – Also known as an *osteopath*, a licensed physician with a doctor of osteopathy or DO degree. May be a general practice physician or a specialist. Osteopathy differs slightly from allopathic medicine in philosophy, but training is practically identical.

**OSTEOPATHIC MANIPULATIVE TREATMENT** – Physical manipulation of a body part as a component of osteopathic treatment.

**OSTEOPOROSIS** – a condition in which the body loses so much bone mass that bones are susceptible to disabling fractures under the slightest trauma

**OSTEOTOMY** – A surgical procedure that involves cutting and repositioning a bone, usually performed in cases of severe joint malalignment

**OVER THE COUNTER** – A term describing drugs or treatments sold without a doctor's prescription.

## P

**PAIN CENTER** – Usually a large medical institution providing comprehensive treatment programs for people in severe or chronic pain.

**PAIN CLINIC** – May be the same as a pain center, but often, a smaller facility offering treatment for people in severe or chronic pain.

**PAIN-MANAGEMENT PLAN** – A comprehensive plan of treatments and strategies designed to help a person manage chronic pain.

**PAIN MEDICINE** – A subspecialty of anesthesiology that focuses on treatment of pain, including chronic and severe acute pain.

**PAIN REHABILITATION** – The process of treating a person in severe or chronic pain and assisting them with developing a long-term plan for managing life with chronic pain.

**PERIPHERAL NERVOUS SYSTEM** – The network of nerves throughout the body that connects the central nervous system (the brain and spinal cord) to organs, blood vessels, muscles, glands and other parts of the body.

**PHYSICAL THERAPIST (PT)** – A licensed health-care professional who specializes in using exercise to treat medical conditions. A PT may prescribe canes and splints. Some are trained in massage and other pain treatments.

**PHYSICAL THERAPY** – Health-care field focusing on exercise and rehabilitation to reduce pain and restore movement following disease, surgery or injury.

**PHYSICIAN ASSISTANT (PA)** – A licensed health-care professional who receives additional training and practices medicine under a physician's supervision, providing patient care, diagnosing illness, offering treatment and, in many states, prescribing drugs for many conditions.

**PILATES** – Exercise technique involving specific postures and stretches designed to strengthen the abdominal muscles.

**PLACEBO EFFECT** – The mysterious phenomenon in which a person receiving an inactive drug or therapy experiences a reduction in symptoms.

**PLANTAR FASCIITIS** – A painful condition in which the thick, fibrous tissue stretching across the sole of your foot, from the heel to the toes, becomes inflamed.

**POLYMYALGIA RHEUMATICA** – a disease causing joint and muscle pain in the neck, shoulders and hips and a general feeling of malaise. The disease is usually marked by a high sedimentation rate (see *erythrocyte sedimentation rate*) and occasionally by a fever.

**POLYMYOSITIS** – An arthritis-related disease in which generalized weakness results from inflammation of the muscles, primarily those of the shoulders, upper arms, thighs and hips. When a skin rash accompanies muscle weakness, the diagnosis is dermatomyositis.

**PRACTITIONER** – A person who performs various alternative or complementary therapies as a vocation or profession.

**PRIMARY-CARE PHYSICIAN** – Doctor who provides general health care to a patient. May be a general practitioner, internist, family physician or osteopath, or may be a pediatrician in the case of a child or adolescent.

**PROLOTHERAPY** – Surgical therapy involving the injection of a chemical irritant into painful soft tissues in order to stimulate blood flow into the affected area and promote pain relief.

**PROSTAGLANDINS** – Hormonelike substances in the body that play a role in pain and inflammation among other body functions.

# Glossary

**PSORIATIC ARTHRITIS** — A form of arthritis that is accompanied by the skin disease psoriasis

**PULSES** – High doses of medicine, such as corticosteroid, provided intravenously.

**PURINE** – One of the two classes of bases involved in the makeup of DNA and RNA; an end-product of purine processing is uric acid. Eating foods rich in purines may contribute to the development of gout; these foods include organ meats, gravies and shellfish.

## Q

**QI GONG** – an Asian practice that incorporates meditation, breathing exercises and movement to promote health and self-healing

## R

**RADIOGRAPH** – X-rays.

**RADIOLOGIST** – Medical doctor who specializes in conducting and examining imaging tests for diagnosis.

**RANGE OF MOTION** – the distance and angles at which your joints can be moved, extended and rotated in various directions

**RAYNAUD'S PHENOMENON** – A condition in which the blood vessels in the hands go into spasms in response to stress or cold temperatures, resulting in pain, tingling and numbness

**RECEPTORS** – The parts of sensory nerves that receive and respond to various stimuli.

**REFERRALS** – When a health-care professional recommends that a patient visit a particular specialist or treatment provider. Referrals may be required by some insurance policies before the patient makes an appointment with the second professional.

**REFILL** – Additional supplies of a prescribed drug dispensed by a pharmacist.

**REFLEX SYMPATHETIC DYSTROPHY** – A chronic pain condition marked by burning pain, swelling and tenderness of an extremity, rising from irritation or damage to nerves in that area. Also known as complex regional pain syndrome.

**REFLEXOLOGY** – Alternative therapy based on a philosophy that applying pressure to particular points on the feet can have an analgesic effect on other, distant parts of the body.

**REM SLEEP** – Stage of sleep marked by "rapid eye movement" in which a person dreams.

**RESECTION** – a surgical procedure that involves removing all or part of a bone, sometimes used to relieve joint pain and stiffness.

**REYE'S SYNDROME** – Dangerous, possibly fatal acute condition associated with the use of aspirin in certain situations, particularly in children. People developing Reye's syndrome may develop swelling of the brain and enlargement of the liver.

**RHEUMATOID ARTHRITIS** – a chronic inflammatory form of arthritis in which the body's otherwise protective immune system turns against the body and attacks tissues of the joints, causing pain, inflammation and deformity.

**RHEUMATOID FACTOR (RF)** – a blood protein (antibody) that is found in high levels in many people with rheumatoid arthritis. It is often associated with RA severity or disease activity, and its presence can be helpful to a doctor in making a diagnosis.

**RHEUMATOLOGIST** – A doctor who specializes in treating arthritis and related diseases, also known as rheumatic diseases. A *pediatric rheumatologist* specializes in treating rheumatic diseases in children.

**ROTATOR CUFF** – A grouping of four tendons that attach to and stabilize the shoulder joints; these tendons can become inflamed and painful through injury or overuse.

## S

**SACROILIAC** – The joints where the spine attaches to the pelvis.

**SALICYLATES** – A subset of NSAIDs derived from salicylic acid, the most common being aspirin. Also refers to topical analgesic ointments containing salicylic acid.

**SCIATICA** – Painful condition involving inflammation of the sciatic nerve, one of the body's largest nerves, which runs from the lower back through the buttocks, with nerve endings extending down the back of the legs to the knees. Sciatica pain is often felt at the back of the thigh.

**SCLERODERMA** – an umbrella term for several diseases that involve the abnormal growth of connective tissue. In most cases, the effects of this overgrowth are limited to the skin and underlying tissues, but in others, tissue

# Glossary

overgrowth can affect the joints, blood vessels and internal organs.

**SED RATE** – see *erythrocyte sedimentation rate*

**SELF-MANAGEMENT** – The process of a person taking an active role in managing his or her own pain or disease, through self-monitoring of health, lifestyle modification, diet, exercise and other means.

**SENSORY NERVES** – Nerves that pick up sensations such as texture, temperature, pressure, pleasure and pain.

**SHIATSU** – Japanese massage technique that is similar to acupressure, but also incorporating stretching techniques.

**SHOCK-WAVE THERAPY** – Alternative therapy involving use of ultrasound technology.

**SOFT-TISSUE RHEUMATIC SYNDROMES** – Painful conditions affecting the soft tissues of the body.

**SOMATIC THERAPY** – In chiropractic philosophy, a treatment method involving a series of special exercises designed to "retrain" the body's muscles, nerves and other organs to move in less painful ways.

**SONOGRAMS** – Images created through ultrasonography or sound-wave technology.

**SPECIALIST** – A physician with additional years of training in a specialized field of medicine. Specialists include orthopaedists, rheumatologists, cardiologists, anesthesiologists, gynecologists and more.

**SPINAL CORD** – Thick cord of nerve tissue that runs from the base of the brain down the spinal canal.

**SPINAL CORD STIMULATION** – Electronic stimulation of the spinal cord through an implanted electronic device as a way to relieve pain.

**SPINAL MANIPULATION** – Physical adjustment of the vertebrae of the spine, particularly in chiropractic or osteopathic treatment.

**SPLINT** – Device used to support or stabilize a joint or to position a joint in a way that prevents further pain or injury to the joint or the soft tissues surrounding it.

**SPONDYLARTHROPATHIES** – a group of arthritis-related diseases that primarily affect the spine

**STEROIDS** – See corticosteroids.

**SUBCUTENAEOUS** – Just beneath the skin. Some medicines are injected subcutaneously, or beneath the skin.

**SUBDERMAL** – Beneath the dermal layer of the skin.

**SUBSTANCE P** – A substance present in the brain believed to be a transmitter of pain impulses.

**SYMPTOM** – Any unusual change in the way a person feels, functions or appears that may indicate disease or injury.

**SYNAPSE** – Gap between nerve cells.

**SYNOVECTOMY** – surgical removal of a diseased joint lining

**SYNOVIAL FLUID** – A slippery liquid secreted by the synovium that lubricates the joint, making movement easier.

**SYNOVIUM** – A thin membrane that lines the joint capsule and can become inflamed (a condition known as synovitis).

**SYNTHETIC** – Manmade or made in a laboratory, as opposed to naturally occurring.

**SYSTEMIC** – A term used to refer to anything that affects the whole body.

## T

**TAI CHI** – an ancient Chinese practice that involves gentle, fluid movements and meditation to help strengthen muscles, improve balance and relieve stress

**TARSAL TUNNEL SYNDROME** – Similar to carpal tunnel syndrome, only involving the nerves of the instep of the foot.

**TENDER POINTS** – Specific, precise areas on the body that are particularly painful upon the application of slight pressure. The finding of tender points is useful in the diagnosis of fibromyalgia.

**TENDER POINT EXAM** – Examination of the patient's tender points to determine diagnosis of fibromyalgia.

**TENDINITIS** – Inflammation of the tendons.

**TENDONS** – Thick connective tissues that attach the muscles to the bones and aid in proper movement.

**TENNIS ELBOW** – A common term for lateral epicondylitis, an inflammation of

# Glossary

the epicondyle, or the area of the bone where the muscles are attached to the elbow.

**TENS** – Transcutaneous electrical nerve stimulation, a treatment for pain that uses a small device to direct mild electric pulses to nerves in a painful area.

**THALAMUS** – The part of the brain where pain messages are first processed.

**THERAPEUTIC DRUGS** – Medications used to treat illness or pain.

**TINNITUS** – Chronic ringing in the ears. Causes vary, including adverse reactions to drugs, injury or infection.

**TOLERANCE** – A gradually developed resistance to the effectiveness of a drug's active ingredients, leading to the need of higher doses of the drug for continued effectiveness.

**TOPHI** – Nodes or masses of crystallized uric acid that settle in various joints in people with gout.

**TRANSDERMAL PATCH** – Small, self-adhering square of plastic that delivers sustained dose of analgesic medication that is absorbed through the skin.

**TRIGGER FINGER** – Stenosing tenosynovitis, a condition involving a thickening of the lining around the tendons in the fingers, causing the finger to lock in a painful, bent position and then to snap open suddenly.

**TUINA** – Chinese massage technique involving manipulation of pressure points.

**TUMOR** – A mass of tissue growth in the body that is distinct from its surrounding structures. May be benign (harmless) or malignant (growing and possibly harmful).

**TUMOR NECROSIS FACTOR** – A cytokine associated with inflammation in rheumatoid arthritis.

## U

**URIC ACID** – Waste product excreted through the kidneys; production of too much uric acid or inadequate excretion of uric acid can lead to gout, where uric acid deposits as crystals in the joint and other tissues.

**URINALYSIS** – Testing of the urine.

## V

**VASCULITIS** – A term describing a group of diseases that involve inflammation of the blood vessels.

**VERTEBRAL SUBLUXATIONS** – In chiropractic philosophy, dislocation or misalignment of the spine that must be adjusted through manipulation.

**VISCOSUPPLEMENTS** – Products injected into osteoarthritis joints (particularly the knee) to replace hyaluronic acid that usually gives the joint fluid its viscosity. Also known as joint fluid therapy.

## W

**WHIPLASH** – Common, painful condition resulting from the neck being whipped back and forth sharply, usually during a fall or accident.

## Y

**YOGA** – A movement practice invented in India and involving a series of body postures called asanas. Yoga incorporates exercise, meditation and breathing components to improve posture and balance, help relieve stress on the joints, and control emotional stress

# Index

# Index

# Index

# Index

# Index

# Index

# Index

# Index

# Index

# Index

# Index

# Trying to Decide Which **Alternative**
# **Treatment** is Right for **You?**

## Find Alternative Treatments That May Work for You!

People with arthritis are among the highest users of alternative therapies, and many have found relief. But some of the products that promise the most offer the least. For the sake of your health and your wallet, you need to know the difference!

Our *Guide to Alternative Therapies* tells you:

- Which nutritional supplements to try – and which to avoid.
- Proven ways to feel better – that won't cost you a cent!
- Ways to bust stress and boost your mood – without side effects.
- What the experts say about alternatives – and how their advice can work for you!

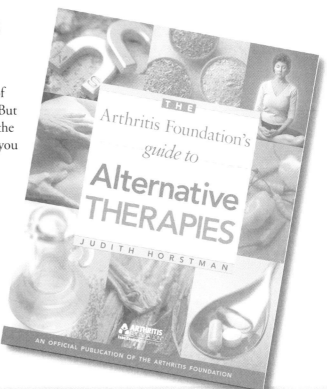

Buy your risk free* copy of *Guide to Alternative Therapies* today for only $24.95.

## To order call (800) 207-8633
## or visit www.arthritis.org

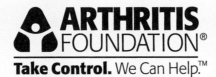

*If any purchase fails to satisfy you, return it within 30 days in its original condition, for a full refund or exchange. Shipping and handling is not refundable.

The Arthritis Foundation has more than 150 local offices across the U.S. To find one near you call (800) 283-7800

CODE0000